# We Endo Warriors

*The Invisible Disease*

Courtney Jetton

*Endo Warriors*
COLLECTIVE

Copyright © 2023 by Courtney Jetton.

All rights reserved. No part of this book may be used or reproduced in any form whatsoever without written permission except in the case of brief quotations in critical articles or reviews.

This book is a memoir. Names, businesses, organizations, places, events and incidents based on real events. Any resemblance to actual persons, living or dead, events, or locales is entirely incidental.

Printed in the United States of America.

For more information, or to book an event, contact :
weendowarriors@gmail.com -
http://www.weendowarriors.com

Book design by Courtney Jetton and Brighton King
Cover design by Courtney Jetton and Brighton King

ISBN-9781666406061
First Edition: October 2023

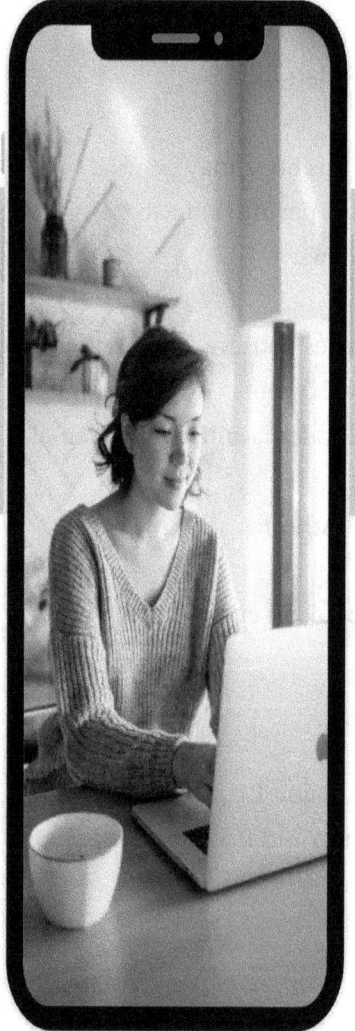

# CONTENTS

WE ENDO WARRIORS ......................................................... I

CONTENTS ............................................................................ I

DEDICATION ........................................................................ 1

INTRODUCTION .................................................................. 2

1 HOW IT BEGAN ................................................................. 9

2 THE DIAGNOSIS ............................................................. 18

3 LIFE WITH ENDOMETRIOSIS ....................................... 31

4 CHELSEA LASCESKI ...................................................... 39

5 CAITLIN MILLER ............................................................ 47

6 KERRY ELLIOT ................................................................ 57

7 MELISSA IRWIN .............................................................. 65

8 STACEY SMITH ............................................................... 79

PART 2 INFERTILITY AND LOSS ..................................... 95

9 ENDOMETRIOSIS AND INFERTILITY ........................ 96

10 IMPACT OF ENDOMETRIOSIS AND INFERTILITY ..... 101

11 THE ULTIMATE FAIL ................................................ 114

12 PERSONAL LESSONS ................................................ 128

**PART 3  FDA AND MEDICAL PROFESSIONALS** ............................................. 137

**13 ENDOMETRIOSIS DESERVES MORE FROM THE FDA** ............................. 138

**14 ENDOMETRIOSOS TREATMENT DEVELOPMENT: THE CHALLENGES OF FDA REGULATION** ................................................................................................ 146

**15 THE LONG ROAD TO DIAGNOSIS: HOW THE MEDICAL SYSTEM FAILS ENDOMETRIOSIS PAITENTS** ............................................................................ 158

**PART 4 DALLAS BUYERS CLUB** ..................................................................... 171

**16 HIV/AIDS AND ENDOMETRIOSIS: DECADES APART BUT STILL FIGHTING THE SAME FIGHT** ............................................................................................ 172

**17 ENDOMETRIOSIS: MISUNDERSTOOD, MISTREATED, MARGINALIZED** ... 190

**18 FIGHTING THE GOOD FIGHT: APPLYING HIV/AIDS ADVOCACY TACTICS TO ENDOMETRIOSIS** ............................................................................................ 206

**PART 5 LACK OF KNOWLEDGE AND AWARNESS** ........................................ 229

**19 THE SILENT SUFFERING: ENDOMETRIOSIS AWARENESS AND THE URGENT NEED FOR EDUCATION** .................................................................................. 230

**20 LOST YEARS OF PAIN: THE LASTING IMPACT OF DELAYED ENDOMETRIOSIS DIAGNOSIS** ..................................................................................................... 237

**21 THE SILENT KILLER: HOW ENDOMETRIOSIS CLAIMS LIVES** ................... 244

**22 ENDOMETRIOSIS AND LOSS OF BODILY AUTONOMY: HOW REPRODUCTIVE RIGHTS AFFECT CHRONIC ILLNESS** .......................................... 256

**PART 6 MEDICATIONS AND TREATMENTS** .................................................. 273

**23 ENDOMETRIOSIS TREATMENT: AN OVERVIEW OF CURRENT OPTIONS TO IMPROVE YOUR LIFE** ..................................................................................... 274

**24 THE HIDDEN DANGERS IN TREATING ENDOMETRIOSIS: WHAT YOUR DOCTOR ISN'T TELLING YOU** ........................................................................ 283

25 ENDING THE SILENCE: GIVING WOMEN WITH ENDOMETRIOSIS A VOICE ............................................................................................................ 290

PART 7 FUNDING AND RESEARCH ........................................................... 298

26 FIGHTING AN INVISIBLE ENEMY: NAVIGATING THE FUNDING MAZE FOR ENDOMETRIOSIS RESEARCH ............................................................ 299

27 ENDOMETRIOSIS FUNDING: WHY THE NEGLECT? ................................ 309

28 THE HIGH PRICE OF ENDOMETRIOSIS: HOW LACK OF RESEARCH FUNDING LIMITS TREATMENT OPTIONS ............................................................ 316

PART 8 ADVOCACY AND ACTION ............................................................. 321

29 ADVOCACY OUTREACH: A CALL TO ACTION FOR ENDOMETRIOSIS AWARENESS ............................................................................................... 322

30 A SYMPHONY OF VOICES: PATIENTS, PROVIDERS AND POLICYMAKERS DRIVING HEALTHCARE REFORM ....................................................... 329

31 WINNING THE ENDOMETRIOSIS BATTLE: A COMPREHENSIVE STRATEGY FOR ADVANCEMENT ............................................................................. 337

32 CONCLUSION .................................................................................... 346

SUMMARY OF KEY POINTS ....................................................................... 349

ABOUT THE AUTHOR ................................................................................ 352

ACKNOWLEDGMENTS ............................................................................... 354

# DEDICATION

In memory of Samuel King, mom and dad love and miss you.
10/15/2022-10/15/2022

Dedicated to all the Endo Warriors living with endometriosis. You are not alone; you are beautiful and strong. Hang in there, you got this!

# INTRODUCTON

Endometriosis is a disorder in which tissue similar to the tissue that lines the uterus grows outside the uterus in places where it does not belong. With endometriosis, deposits of tissue that act just like the tissue lining the uterus develop outside the uterus (World Health Organization: WHO & World Health Organization: WHO, 2023). This tissue thickens, breaks down, and bleeds with each period. The blood has nowhere to go and is then reabsorbed and more lesions form, the process repeats.

The cause of endometriosis is unknown, however; there is speculation that birth control from a young age, the excessive amounts of estrogen, or even genetics are to blame. There is no known cure or preventative for endometriosis. However, the symptoms may be individually treated.

Endometriosis causes a chronic inflammatory reaction that attacks the entire body. The formation of scar tissue as a result of burst adhesions and fibroids often occurs.

There are different forms of adhesions to include: superficial endometriosis found on the pelvic peritoneum, cystic ovarian endometriosis found on the ovaries, deep endometriosis found in the recto-vaginal septum, bladder, and bowel, and in can be found on surrounding organs and imbedded in muscle tissue outside the pelvic area.

Endometriosis has a significant impact on all aspects of women's lives who live with this debilitating disease. It decreases quality of life due to severe pain, fatigue, depression, anxiety, and infertility. Many women are unable to work or do basic daily tasks due to the severity of their endometriosis. Relationships often are affected by endometriosis by painful intercourse, avoidance, misunderstanding, and more.

By giving women with endometriosis a voice, we are allowing them the opportunity to be heard. Advocating for awareness and funding to further research and understand endometriosis will benefit women living with endometriosis. Women are misdiagnosed and ignored by medical professionals more often than one may think. We are often told there is no reason for the pain that they can find and treat us as if it is all in our heads. It takes at least 10-13 years for a proper diagnosis as things stand today. Even still, due to the overwhelming lack of awareness and understanding women are consistently losing their jobs, relationships, and livelihood to endometriosis. Medical professionals refuse to listen or acknowledge women living with endometriosis, leaving them feeling hopeless and even more alone in the fight against endometriosis. [1]

Moving forward through this book we will visit topics such as personal stories from myself and others around the nation and world, discuss infertility and loss and talk about the FDA and medical professionals. We will discuss the correlations between the movie Dallas Buyers Club and fighting endometriosis today. The book further goes to talk about lack of knowledge and

---

[1] World Health Organization: WHO & World Health Organization: WHO. (2023). Endometriosis. www.who.int. https://www.who.int/news-room/fact-sheets/detail/endometriosis#:~:text=Key%20facts,age

awareness, medications and treatments, funding, and research, and lastly advocacy and action.

*"As a kid I had bad periods. Horrible debilitating pain that would make you throw up, severe cramps, unregulated periods, blood clots, and sometimes would bleed for weeks instead of just 7 days; would bleed so bad that I would flood every and anything I would wear. I heard of endometriosis growing up but didn't know what it really was until I had my own daughter.*

*Growing up she was a healthy 135-140 pound kid that loved the outdoors and was in the Blazers at school, active in soccer growing up and was happy and healthy. When she turned into a teenager, that's when her bad periods started, I thought yeah, she's taking after me and would give her the same things I took as a teen. Took her to the doctor and put her on birth control at age 14 to regulate her periods...that did not work. We would buy the super flow tampons and pads and many months she would go through the whole box, and all the pads.*

*Her senior year of high school we notice her losing her weight, a little at first, we thought maybe she is losing her baby fat. Really didn't pay much attention to it. After school she went through a hard period in her life and lost a ton of weight due to stress, and that is what we chalked it up to. Then she made the decision to get married, by this time she wasn't even 100 pounds, still having horrible periods, not eating. We still thought it was stress and not eating due to the stress. She got pregnant with our grandson and that is when I heard she had endometriosis, still did not really know much about it, because doctors never really talk about it; they do not explain anything to you as a patient to family member. I had to hear from co-workers how it can spread to other parts of the body. You are basically helpless. She had a very rough pregnancy and barely gained any weight, but she did give birth to P man. Years later she did, however, lose a child due to the endo; one of the side effects of endo are blood clots. One developed in the umbilical cord, and we lost our baby grandson, due to endo. The doctor wanted to dismiss a blood clot when I told him that is what caused it, and he said he did not think that is what happened.... until he saw it. It is very heartbreaking for a mother to see her child go through everything and there is nothing you can do to make it go away or even make it better.*

# We Endo Warriors

*My daughter is in her late 20's now and is sick, sick of being sick, sick of doctors who are unwilling to help her. She is tired of feeling sick, tired and in pain all the time. I know doctors say is "try this try that...," no, she needs real help and if you do not have the right insurance or the right amount of money then you're stuck, and they put you off. Endo is not talked about to women. The options are not there for women to make choices for their own bodies. Men doctors have no clue because they are men and, do not go through things females go through. If you're lucky you find a female doctor that has endo and can relate, but not all women have endo. With all my history with my periods I have never had endo.*

*My daughter weighs less than 100 pounds and is not healthy, she is in constant pain and every time you turn around she's bleeding. All I can tell her is call her doctor when she's hurting and in so much pain, hoping she will, and they can give her something at least for the pain. These doctors need to listen to their patients and do what they ask, it's their bodies and they know what they go through every day, instead of ignoring them and putting them off. Endo is real and I have seen the effects it has and the outcome of having endo." – Marissa Webb*

# PART 1

## PERSONAL EXPERIANCES

## 1

## HOW IT BEGAN

I reflect on my childhood and remember how much I dreaded going to school. I hated middle school so much. It was about sixth grade when I realized that something was wrong with me, but I did not understand what or how. I just knew I was sick all the time and calling home every day for headaches and cramps. The school has rules on going to the restroom and being out of class during class hours, I would bleed through my uniform and be forced to wear my hoodie around my waist. One, the teachers would not let you out of class, and two, my mom got to where she thought I was just trying to get out of school.

As time went on, mom started to realize that something was indeed very wrong. She went toe to toe with the principle over their ridiculous bathroom rules and to allow girls to go to the rest room whenever they asked, no questions asked. As we needed to freedom to be able to take care of ourselves. Better yet, schools really should have complementary feminine hygiene products in their bathrooms. I remember during that time that many of us were just getting our cycle, many girls did not have access to those products, and we had to share our products our moms got us with the girls who did not have any. Many times, we would run out during the day and had to ask anyone and everyone if they happened to have a spare tampon or pad.

In the beginning, I remember over all just being extremely uncomfortable. Heavy bleeding and some rough cramps. The gynecologist at the time just chocked it up to simply – heavy bleeding and bowel pain – as if it were constipation or something.

# We Endo Warriors

*"That's just bowel movements, that's normal."*

I was 13 years old, and it was my first time speaking to him alone without Mom in the room. The first experience I can recall being blown off by a medical professional. Provided I have been seeing this man since I was 10 or 11 when Mother Nature first presented her lovely gift to me. Mom had always gone in with me up until I turned thirteen and went into my annual check.

Looking back, I reflect on how fast everyone was to throw me on birth control. We tried every form of pill there was available at the time trying to combat the heavy bleeding. Even went as far as trying to stop the cycle for several months at a time. Now as we all know, this obviously affects your hormones, more so than they already are messed up naturally. The goal was to attempt to balance them. At the time, I was what I consider to be a "Yes Woman." I agreed to anything and everything that doctor suggested to me, I was in my early teens and desperate for relief of some kind. I was tired of bleeding for months on end with no end in sight. I will be the first to admit that this one birth control Seasonique® was my favorite thing. Cycle free for three months at a time

I stayed on Seasonique® all the way up till I turned 18 years old and graduated school. I went through a period in high school where I was once super athletic and healthy, I struggled from time to time, but nothing compared to what was about to happen to me. Freshman year was a breeze, I was a part of JROTC and of the Blazer Adventure Team. I was good at it too, successful, happy. Then the summer between Freshman and Sophomore year hit. I went from 130 pounds to barley 100 pounds. I recall mom thinking I was on drugs and giving me pregnancy test every week it felt like.

Of course, the test was always negative, cause contrary to popular believe, I was the good kid. The whole drug assumption deal along with the massive weight loss and vomiting led to many, many doctors' visits over the next few years. Lots of blood work and testing, and nothing ever showed up. This then led to being accused and suspected on bulimia. Boy, that phase of life was loads of fun. Not. I grew more and more tired all the time, my motivation for the things I loved, like Blazers fizzled out. Everything was becoming bothersome and more of a burden. I just wanted to lay in bed and be left alone. I remember, that lead to loads of trouble for myself.

My parents were forcing me to eat, trying to put me on protein diets and such. I continued to get sick and really could not help it. It was embarrassing, even more embarrassing to be accused of drug use, bulimia, you name it. Now it is not my parents' fault for thinking this. I did not have the words to describe what was really going on, as I did not even know this was all cycle related and considered abnormal. I just knew I felt awful all the time and bled constantly. I used to resent my parents for a long time for the way I felt like I was being treated.

Ultimately, during junior year my interest in all my favourite things started dyeing out. I honestly was just too tired. Every time we went to run out to the field or workout, I was having personal complications of my own. Which in that ACU uniform was difficult to hide. I figured out that layering clothes helped. I cannot count how many times we went on an FTX what I ended up chafing and bleeding during. The combination was hell. These things had been going on since the beginning of being on Blazers, however; eventually you get tired. That and cramping all the time, I genuinely just felt horrible 24/7. Could not tell anyone that though, cause then you are just trying to get out of whatever it is that is going on.

Senior year I completely dropped out of all my extracurriculars. My team resented me for it too. To reiterate, I just did not enjoy it anymore. Running and heavy work outs just lead to bleeding through my ACUs, and I resented that. I do not remember a lot from senior year at all. I want to say that senior year when I was eighteen was the last of my normal life as I knew it. I still stayed sick all the time, that just became a part of my daily life.

Visiting home usually resulted in comments about how sickly I looked and speculation of drug use. I had to learn to just ignore them, they do not live in my body.

Later, in 2016 I got married and in November of 2016, we learned we were pregnant. At this point in when life decided to take a huge turn for the worst. That pregnancy was rough to say the least. I was all of ninety-four pounds through majority of the experience and was on a protein shake diet for a good portion of the time. Again, this was before the diagnosis came. Pregnancy was hard on my body; I struggled the entire time. In and out of the ER being sent to Labor and Delivery every time I turned around. I hit that 22-week mark and my body decided it was not about that pregnant life anymore.

Fortunately, my son is strong and hardheaded. Every week was a waiting game, I was put on bed rest and the whole nine yards. Now anyone who has been forced on bed rest knows that it is difficult to stay in bed like that. My mother-in-law was on me all the time for being up messing around with animals or saving kittens. (Yes, I am that person to go under houses to retrieve a stray crying kitten at 7 months pregnant. The hole was the perfect size for me to fit through and not even touch my belly.)

Between the struggle with weight gain, anemia, horrific pain, nausea, and my body constantly trying to go into labour since the 22-week mark it became a very exhausting battle. When it came time to have our son, I was 36-weeks along. I had been in labor for a few days and did not know. The pain just felt like normal everyday pain to me even outside of pregnancy. So, it did not occur to me that anything was different. It only became evident when my hips were so uncomfortable that I would squat just to find relief. My mother-in-law timed my contractions and off we went to the hospital.

Turned out my water had had a slow leak for a few days. I did not have that movie scene gush of water everyone knows about. They went in and popped it manually the rest of the way. I agreed to take the epidural, which a later decided I would never do again, should the question come up again. After a little bit of a stressful delivery our little boy Parrish was born June 10, 2017, at 2:04 PM. It took a nurse pushing down on my stomach and help from a few others to get him unstuck. It was like as soon as it came time to push all the contractions suddenly stopped. It felt like eternity. He ended up having to go to the NICU for a week because of jaundice.

# We Endo Warriors

I was one of them fortunate souls who got to keep their pre-pregnancy body. In my case however, this was deadly. I have a photo somewhere of myself holding my son, dark circles under my eyes, bones clearly visible in my face, shoulders, and arms. I was deathly ill and severely underweight. The post-partum doctor, immediately set me up with a dietitian. Whom I have only met the one time. Her words are forever burned into my soul, "You are sick, you're smaller than my daughter who weighs 110 pounds; If you keep going down this path you will die.".

*"You are sick, you're smaller than my daughter who weighs 110 pounds; If you keep going down this path you will die."*

My husband spent a lot of time trying to cook up the heartiest high protein meals of which he could think. Which consisted of red meats, potatoes, salads, you know the kind. To no avail, I was still unable to gain weight. I reached back up to 104 and just sat there for the next several years.

# 2

## THE DIAGNOSIS

It was not till several years after I had my son that I got diagnosed, October 2019. It took several doctors, several attempts at finding help, many emergency room visits and the list goes on before I found one man who was willing to listen and help. He was the only soul who seemed genuinely concerned. Just so happened that mom had been using him the last several years, since our original guy retired. You know the one, previously mentioned. My doctor was a Godsend, he and his team were phenomenal. They even knew about my husband when he wrecked his bike and was hospitalized at a separate hospital in the next town over and would ask about his well-being when I visited. My husband and I ended up having surgery on the same day, October 11th, 2019, in two separate towns.

The whole reason I ended up in this new doctors' care was because my mom had been doing her research and suggested I investigate this disease called Endometriosis. What's Endometriosis? I wondered. After doing the good ole Google search it was what really matched my symptoms from the past 10 years. That little generic definition of what Endometriosis was at the time fit the bill. Back then, it was in its beginning phases of spreading like a monster.

Pregnancy and childbirth really mad it angry and it hit vigorously. Endometriosis is said to only been seen via laparoscopic surgery. At least that is what I have been told and have read several times over. Depending on where you look you may find some women stating it could be found via MRI. I just know that first surgery that led to my diagnosis after 13 long years of begging and pleading with anyone that might could listen, was a laparoscopic laser surgery. They had gone in, discovered proof of Endometriosis, took biopsies of it and lasered everything they could find at the time.

I had endometrial lesions behind my colon, and severe scar tissue if I remember correctly. Bear in mind this was October of 2019, two years after having my first child and what I consider to be the forefront of what was soon to come. My doctor made the argument that all those years of being on birth control from a young age was the cause. Stating that my hormones never really got the chance to level themselves out, we also discussed the abundance of the hormone estrogen being a possible culprit. All of this in speculation of course.

I later learned that they do not really understand Endometriosis, where it comes from, how it happens, what causes it to even occur. The statement made was, "There just isn't enough research on it, it's a fairly new disease."

*"There just isn't enough research on it, it's a fairly new disease."*

As a form of hormonal therapy, they had implanted the copper wire IUD during that surgery. To help balance that excessive estrogen that was speculated to be the culprit and to help lessen the periods. Boy, the trouble that thing gave me. I went two years with it and steady was getting sicker and sicker, the pain was steady getting worse. Especially on my left side. Literally felt like my left ovary was exploding. It had migrated in implanted into the left side of my uterine wall. After going to the ER for pain, and not being helped, nor my doctor accepting me back because I owed him money after my surgery that my lovely insurance company decided not to cover, I ended up pulling that IUD out myself.

**DO NOT go pulling out your IUD yourself. That is a no-no.**

That was a horrible experience, painful and nauseating. I sat in the tub for hours vomiting my guts up. I cried and pleaded with whatever entity was listening begging for the strength to do it and follow through with it. Pleading to God to make this all end, asking why I was dealt such an awful deck of cards in my life. I was completely aware of the risk I was taking. But I did not care, I was desperate for relief.

I did it though, it felt awful dislodging it from that left wall but boy did the pressure and pain immediately cease and I took a huge sigh of relief. Cried even with happiness. I think that night I slept in peace for the first time in a long time since having that thing put in. Since then, I have refused anything they have suggested. I have done learned my lesson.

I did end up going back to the ER with the IUD in hand and telling them what I had done and why. I also told them that the doctor refused to see me due to a money issue with the insurance refusing to cover the remaining cost. To which they firstly looked horrified and secondly, looked at me like a heathen because I could not afford it pay such an outrageous bill at the time. They also treated me as drug seeking.

I just laughed at them at this point, you get past a point of being upset and freaking out, to a point where you just get straight angry and decide you do not have time for their games anymore. It is a combination of feeling hopeless and a strong disdain. Depending on who you are your anger may come out differently, but I laugh and shake my head, often telling them how useless they are and how they need to really educate themselves.

Eventually you become a bit bitter towards, medical professionals, you get to where you refuse at all costs to ever go back to the ER or to a doctor with your problems because you already know the inevitable, they will not help you.

I have tried Orilissa® as well. At the time it was a relatively new drug being tested to treat Endometriosis pain. It was $2,000 without insurance for a 3-month pack. I certainly could not afford that, my doctor had to fight with insurance to cover it, let alone the surgery. It made me angry that the same insurance company covered nearly 100% of my husband's surgeries surrounding his motorcycle accident but it was a battle for them to cover what I needed.

Orilissa® was okay, it took the edge off but really did not help. I often wondered why I was even taking this drug if it was not helping. The doctor just said to give it time. The problem with that was that I do not particularly like taking pills for any excessive amount of time. I hate taking pills as it is. I do not want my body to become dependent on these experimental drugs or any drug for that matter to just function from day to day.

Yes, some form of pain relief would be great, something stronger maybe on a as needed basis. Not something that has got to be taken multiple times a day religiously. We often get addressed and treated as 'drug seeking,' I do not even think we are looking for medicinal help, we are simply looking for some genuine answers to make life more liveable and comfortable: a cure. It is so frustrating to be treated as drug seeking when you do not even have a drug like past.

Eventually, I just gave up all together. I just dealt with it. I got to where I would find comfort in hot baths and laying down whenever possible. I just got to where I would not do much more than basic housework and raising my son. This affected my marriage greatly. Our marriage was already going downhill due to my own

# We Endo Warriors

lack thereof within the marriage. Sex, physical contact of any kind, tempers flaring, misunderstanding the whole nine yards.

He [2]and I simply could never see eye to eye. He did not understand me. He thought I was just lazy or being a baby about things, or that I did not want him anymore. I was dying inside; the pain was gradually getting worse. Sex was painful, physical touch is painful, sometimes just breathing and moving is painful. Not to mention the nonstop excessive bleeding. It never stopped, ever. It gets to a point where your spouse truly gets fed up with you being sick all the time and cutting into their lives with your nonsense. Your become a burden, a problem for those around you.

---

[2] For stats on how endometriosis affects partners:

Ameratunga, D., Flemming, T., Angstetra, D., Ng, S.-K., & Sneddon, A. (2017). Exploring the impact of endometriosis on partners. *Journal of Obstetrics and Gynaecology Research, 43*(6), 1048-1053. Retrieved 6 18, 2023, from https://ncbi.nlm.nih.gov/pubmed/28621048

At family gatherings, when you come up in topic it is like all anyone has to say about you is that your lazy, and sick all the time. Your skinny and sickly and the gossip about potential drug use gets thrown around. You become a shell of a person, way off deep into depression, miserable and unhappy. It gets to where you wish it would all end. This disease really sends you into some dark places mentally. All we really want is relief and a normal life.

I do not really believe such a thing exists. This life really seems hopeless much of the time. I would not go as far as feeling suicidal, but feeling like you wished it would all just stop and go away, just wishing for a different body would best describe where I was. I was just empty inside, alone and in a dark place. I lived there for a long time by myself. My marriage really was not the main cause but still was not as healthy or supportive as it should have been. We ultimately separated in February of 2021. It was a clean separation no bad blood; however, we did get into a disagreement once and the thing he said to me still rings in my mind today. He said, "Good luck finding anyone to put up with you, you don't even put out!"

# We Endo Warriors

I have read in Endo support groups that many women with Endo hear those very words. Gradually over the years I started to defend myself and learn that I really do not owe anyone an explanation, especially if they cannot even take the time to understand my life even remotely or how my body works. Much less respect me.

I do not hold anything against him. I just have not forgotten. The insults that come with living with endometriosis are endless, especially if you end up surrounding yourself with the wrong people. It just stems from misunderstanding and lack of knowledge. They do not know any better, many never will. You must remove stressors from your life, stressing does not help and will send you right back into a flair up.

I spent a lot of time trying to rebuild my life and trying to narrow down my stressors. It was not until I met Alex that I truly began to learn about endometriosis from a new perspective. Alex really has been the most amazing partner to go through this with. He does his research and is constantly looking up holistic ways of combating endometriosis. This was really the first time in my life that anyone outside of my mom has taken a real interest or concern into my health and wellbeing. He does not judge me or make me feel bad for how my life is. He has been an apart of trying to find a solution, and no number of words can describe how thankful I am for him.

With Alex doing research and teaching me about holistic medicine, we have been able to try simple things such as alkaline diets, and Heal-All tinctures or teas. We have learned that our systems being overly acidic will cause inflammation and swelling. We have learned that there are natural, healthy ways to manage endometriosis that do not require harsh medicines from medical providers. Alex has been a blessing in my life and is one of the major factors making this book possible for all of you today.

What peaked Alex's interest into the disease was when my brother was living with me, and he had told Alex that he was scared and never wanted me to do it again. He is referring to the week I spent in the bathroom floor both bleeding out and vomiting. Quite sure he even walked in on me and was horrified, as he was the very first person to really witness first-hand what endometriosis looked like.

Alex then sat me down and we had a lengthy conversation about why it was important for me to talk to people and be very honest with them, no matter how disgusting or uncomfortable it might be for both parties. As Alex believes that in doing so, people will not be scared when they walk in on it, and two, people may better understand why I behave the way I do about certain things. He was also referring to how to better handle employers when I would have to call in to work or rush to an ER.

Alex taught me that my health, for myself and my son, far outweighs the need to be at work. If I do not take care of myself properly, I would be no use at work anyway. He taught me to not feel bad for putting myself first for once. It was tricky when I did start trying to implement his words into my life. I have made a lot of people angry by putting myself and my health before the needs of others for a change. He was 100% right though, I absolutely had to take better care of myself and fight back.

# 3

## LIFE WITH ENDOMETRIOSIS

Living with this disease has been the most exhausting thing in my life. I am tired all the time, like extreme exhaustion. The pain associated with endometriosis is out of this world. Each woman may describe her pain differently from the next, but in my case this pain far exceeds that of child labor or any other pain I have experienced in life. It is like child labor times 100. It makes my body feel heavy like wet cement, my organs feel hot like literal lava running through my veins, my hips and lower back hurt so bad it is hard to move most days. On especially difficult days I have extreme pain shooting down my right leg to the point it is difficult to walk, much less move. Sometimes even under my ribs and mid to upper back, shoulders and neck are super stiff and sore. Migraines are often another additional gift this disease presents itself with.

I had to do a project for college once that was something about drawing out how you would visualize endometriosis as if describing it to a friend. I remember I drew a uterus, red and inflamed, engulfed in flames, lava and wrapped in barbed wire. I added little black lesions and blood seeping from the lesions. Let us just say that was a particularly rough day. It led to a large group discussion about what Endometriosis is and basically just arguing your general generic Google description against my real-life experience.

I constantly feel guilty thinking about my children. I wish I could be that cool mom that does everything with them. Jumping on the trampoline, rough housing, running, working out with our oldest boy. I just cannot anymore, I move the wrong way I am bleeding profusely and swelling up. Lift something heavy? Not even all that heavy and I am bleeding profusely and swelling. I used to be a dog groomer. I would even say that in the beginning I was a sharp groomer, but as time went on, my skills waned and my desire and enjoyment for the job went out the window.

You could tell in my work my heart was not in it anymore. Not because I dislike it, no, because I was in constant agony and suffering in silence and it just became unenjoyable. You see, your employers do not see what is going on. All they see and perceive is someone who has probably become lazy and hates their job. I know this to be fact because I often read the client comments on Facebook when I would take off or take a break from grooming talking about what useless help I was to my employer. I had read that "There isn't any good, reliable help anymore," or something like "Again?!, You need to find someone better."

My employer sure gave me their fair share of grief about life as well. I do not even really blame them. I mean, how could someone possibly understand the truth if they cannot see for themselves what is happening? I do not know how many times I would try my best to hide the fact I was running off to the restroom to get sick due to a nauseating amount of pain. Or buying boxes upon boxes of tampons each time I ran over to the dollar store for lunch.

Eventually, we did end up discussing the problem, however; that just leads to "I'm cramping and I'm here every single day." I remember thinking to myself, girl, we are nowhere near on the same ball field here. I can recall the pure resentment I felt reading that text while I was laid out on my bathroom floor, both bleeding out all over the place and vomiting my guts up. I attempted to take a shower; even though that was such a major task that I had practically fallen out of the shower next to the toilet and just laid there for the rest of the day.

I remember, after I had my first son, I had noticed a few new additional abnormal things happening to me. I would be standing next to his crib, changing his diaper or something when out of nowhere a huge gush of blood came out of nowhere and covered my white floors. Thank sweet baby Jesus for tile. Mind you, my son was about 8 months old in this instance. So, this was not postpartum leftovers. I cannot recall if there was any major alarming pain associated outside of what my normal was at the time. I just remember cleaning up gigantic messes all the time. I remember feeling scared and wondering what it was. Miscarriage crossed our minds, which was not the case though. Pregnancy does not come easy for me.

I cannot count the days and nights; I would just let my son play in the bathroom floor while I just laid in the tub with the shower running and just bleeding so much that it was simply better to lay in the shower till it let up. The endless days of lying in bed with massive migraines and never being too far from the restroom. My dad was staying with us at the time, and I really did try to hide what my life really was like. I have always hidden the worst parts of my life from my family, even my husband. As I mentioned previously, my brother was the first to witness the reality of the disease many years later in 2021 when he was living with me.

I still live life scoping out restaurants and peoples' homes for the nearest restroom should an event occur. I still have severe migraines, excessive pain that never seems to go away, constantly going through the cycle of bad and good days. Endometriosis is not just heavy periods and bad cramps. It irks me so much when I hear that.

Endometriosis is hell. It behaves like a cancer yet is not a cancer. It is painful, so painful it puts childbirth to shame; at least for me. Pain is so nauseating that any movement either triples your migraine or makes you throw up, many times it does both. Sometimes it is an all over body experience. It attacks the entire immune system. Painful bowel movements and urination, the inflammation is hard core when we have flair ups.

It attacks your nervous system, muscular system, endocrine system, the list goes on. The disease is quite invasive. It far exceeds the reproductive system. It has been seen to cause infertility, miscarriage, and loss. I would even go as far as saying stillbirths are even in question. If it can cause infertility and miscarriage, why wouldn't it be a link to some stillbirths? It is not unreasonable to think so, regardless of what medical professionals may tell you. Remember these are the same folks letting us go ten plus years undiagnosed and refusing to believe us anyway. I do not hold much merit to what any of them have to say anymore.

Endometriosis is severe migraines, weight loss, or weight gain depending on the woman, hair loss, mental health struggles, extreme exhaustion; absolutely zero energy. Painful intercourse, overall, I personally find touch in general very painful during a flair up. Flair ups consist of extreme bloating, excessive heavy bleeding, nausea, debilitating pain, diarrhea or constipation, painful urination.

---

## **Symptoms List**

- Heavy Bleeding
- Extreme Pain ALL OVER
- Constipation or Diarrhea
- Painful Urination
- Bloating
- Hair loss
- Weight Gain/Loss
- Mental Health Decline
- Attacks Entire Immune System
- Spreads Outside of just the reproductive area
- Nausea/ Constantly Getting and Staying Sick
- Infertility, Miscarriage and Loss

- Burning Sensations
- Feeling Heavy like wet cement
- Sometimes Breaking Out in Rashes
- Extreme Exhaustion
- Migraines
- Lightheadedness
- Dizziness
- Fainting Spells
- No Energy for days/months on end
- Bleeding outside of the period
- Bleeding for days/months on end
- Painful Intercourse
- Immune System Disorder[3]

---

[3] Information taken from The Mayo Clinic and taken from other Endo Warriors

# 4

## CHELSEA LASCESKI

I have always had extremely painful periods, but doctors would not listen to me. They just told me it was bad periods; everyone has one, what do you think they should feel like, etc. From the time I was in my teens. I was given birth control after birth control with awful side effects and no help.

When I first went to the gyno at 16, they told me I had Dysmenorrhea and he put me on a birth control pill. I tried it for three months and just felt sick all the time and it did not help. They gave me another pill option with the same effects. I did that for four different types of pills. Then I had a switch in doctors (mine left), and he wanted me to get the IUD. I was reluctant but tried it and it was the longest 9 months of my life.

I bled almost 24/7, had horrible cramps, and ended up having to have it removed due to crazy amounts of blood and migrating. During this time, I was prescribed Naproxen®. My final try was the NuvaRing®. It did help a little bit but then insurance stopped covering it, so I had to stop it. All throughout this process my doctors kept telling me that I was just being dramatic, all women have periods, just get pregnant and that will help, I just need to learn to deal with it, etc.

I then just accepted this as my life and that I was just a wuss with pain. I genuinely thought I just had an extremely low pain tolerance. Apparently passing out, vomiting, and being in debilitating pain was normal. Then a few years ago my one week a month of terrible pain started creeping into two weeks. Not only was my period debilitating but ovulation time was also causing a lot of pain. Then I started not being able to manage with ibuprofen as well as before. The pain was breaking though much stronger and making it much harder to function.

Then in December 2021 I was in so much pain and bleeding so heavy I could barely function. I was having roughly five good days a month at this point. I went to a new doctor in January 2022, and she said, "I think you have endometriosis,", but still only wanted to treat me with either Orilissa® or depo shot or my favorite, "just get pregnant". I refused the shot and reluctantly tried Orilissa®. I was on it for almost three months, and it was awful, and I stopped taking it. I had so many issues and side effects from it. I still had pain and bleeding, I was getting debilitating pain every afternoon, losing hair, joint pain, depression, not feeling like myself (it is so hard to describe but I just was not me).

*"I think you have Endometriosis."*

I had called and asked to stop it multiple times explaining my symptoms only to be told to just give it some time. Finally, it got so bad I could not get up from the floor and I called and said they must tell me how to safely stop or I am just going to quit on my own. I could not do it anymore. I had now been to the ER a few times for debilitating pain only to be told that everything was fine. They would give me pain meds and fluids and send me home. My gyno finally sent me a referral to a specialist after my amazing ER doctor sent notes from my visit to her explaining this cannot keep going on; I could not get into the specialist for 10 months.

I tried to just manage symptoms with my Primary Care Physician until my specialist appointment but realized after losing almost 50lbs in a very short time due to not being able to eat or keep things down, so many ER trips I can't keep track, continued decline in my health, and my increasing pain that I wasn't going to make it until my appointment. It was in august of 2022 while getting ready to go back to school and realizing I was still about 5 months away that I knew I needed to do something. I desperately searched for a different specialist that I could see sooner. I found a doctor and within a month I had an appointment. September 1st, I met with the PA, and she instantly told me I needed to meet with the surgeon.

This was an urgent case he needed to see. September 30th, I met with the surgeon. He looked at me and told me "This is not in your head, your pain is real, and I'm going to help you." I had been having some major blood pressure and heart issues, so I needed cardiac clearance before I was able to have surgery. During that time, I found out I have POTS. I was then finally able to have safe surgery where I was diagnosed with stage 4 Endometriosis, covering everything in November 2022. I was told I must have 6 months of hormone treatment to put me into menopause before I can have excision surgery. My specialist said it is too dangerous to do surgery without this treatment.

*"This is not in your head, your pain is real, and I'm going to help you."*

I reluctantly did the Zoladex® implant in the beginning of January 2023, but my body did not handle it well. I had many physical side effects and depression was scary. My only choice was to go ahead with the surgery because I was told it was unsafe to continue or try anything else. January was rough; February landed me in the ER more times than I can count, and by March 2023, I was fighting for my life while waiting for my surgery on April 3rd. I had a scary surgery where Endometriosis was excised from all over and five cysts and endometriomas were removed.

If my doctors had listened to me earlier maybe I would not be completely covered in this awful disease. Maybe I would not have lost so much to this! I feel like this disease has taken everything from me and I do not feel like I even exist anymore. This disease is so much more than physical pain. The mental pain that comes with this is unreal! So many dark days and even darker nights where I could not see the light at the end of the tunnel. So many nights I prayed for it to just end because the pain was so bad and no end in sight; wishing that I never woke up. Pain makes you desperate and think things you cannot imagine.

The loneliness of this disease, the guilt that comes with not being able to do things you want or need to do, the feeling of being a failure and broken; like you are not enough, like you have died and been replaced with someone who cannot function. Losing friendships, jobs, missing things because you do not feel well enough, etc. So many tears, feeling like such a burden, and just not feeling ok. Financially it is also extremely difficult because I cannot work all the time, have medical bills, extras needed to function, on top of normal living expenses.

---

Chelsea's story is just one of many. The struggle to get help is insane. The lack of compassion from medical professionals is proving repeatedly to be a problem. The amount of time it takes from first having problems to finally being diagnosed is simple unacceptable. The average amount of time it takes to finally be diagnosed is roughly 10 years. Only after having very birth control known to man thrown at, you, and shoved down your throat. The fact that we are led to believe that the pain, bleeding, and symptoms we experience are normal.

Chelsea mentions a great point here talking about the financial burden endometriosis brings to our lives. The medical bills, the hundreds of dollars every month spent on feminine products or clothing because of uncontrollable bleeding, the money that goes into medicine or heating pads and so on and so forth. The list is never ending. Endometriosis in its more severe forms will impact our jobs and livelihoods. At which point we are losing money, thus losing access to funding for food, bills, our homes, and so much more.

# 5

## CAITLIN MILLER

Everyone has painful craps on their period, as a 10-year-old who just started their period the pain was horrible. I just felt horrible, and my period lasted so long and was so heavy; we began contraceptives a few months after my first period, which helped.

I was an active member at school. I played basketball, ran for student council, and did band. However, on July 7th, 2019, not even two months after my 16th birthday my little brother's babysitter woke me up to come stay downstairs with my brother and lock the door behind her as she left for work. I woke up in extreme pain and was very nauseous and just felt like I needed to go to the bathroom. So, I followed her to the front of the house and locked the door behind her, going into our bathroom right beside my brother's room.

I immediately sat down thinking I needed to poop and after trying for a few minutes I immediately felt hot and sick to my stomach. I sat on the edge of the tub beside the toilet and let my head dangle, I began to feel lightheaded and was burning up. I decided to take my chance on our cold tile floor. I laid down on the floor and immediately grabbed my stomach as it felt like I had just gone 6 rounds with Freddy from Nightmare on Elm Street. I began to cry and whimper but my mom could not hear me. Suddenly, I heard buzzing thinking I had left my phone upstairs by my bed. I used every bit of energy to reach for it in every twist I felt like giving up but luckily, I told myself - one more shot - and was able to grab it. It was the babysitter's husband calling to make sure she made it to work, I answered with tears streaming down my face and my voice cracking.

Immediately he knew something was wrong and called my mom to wake her up, letting her know I was in pain.

My mom rushed into the bathroom and found me on the floor, asking me repeatedly, "What is wrong?", as I had to tell her I do not know. Eventually she decided to take me to the ER, waking my dad up to come, lift me off the floor and get into her car. We rushed to the hospital where I do not remember sitting in the waiting room long, but I do remember lying in the bed and being taken away for so many tests.

My supervisor at the time kept calling my phone and told me since I was a no-call no-show I would no longer have a job, hospital or not. I did not care; I just wanted the pain to stop and the fear in my mom's eyes to go away. Repeatedly the doctor would come in giving me more and more painkillers that were not helping at all. Continuously my mom was being pulled out of the room and asked if I was a substance abuser by the doctor on shift, finally there was a shift change. A new doctor came in, read my file, saw I was still in pain and decided to run 2-3 more tests. He immediately pulled my mom out of the room; I was scared as a 16-year-old,

I had no idea what was going on and the pain felt like I should have been dead hours before.

Finally, my mom returns to my room and tells me with tears in her eyes that I am going into emergency surgery. I, a 16-year-old, needing emergency surgery; I thought what in the hell is going on? I am immediately prepared for surgery before my mom can even call my dad and let him know what's going on. I later found out that I had an exceptionally large cyst on my ovary which burst and was causing me to bleed internally. During surgery, my doctor noticed small dark spots on the abdominal wall, telling my mom it was extremely important to follow up with my OB/GYN to find out what it was. He had suspicions that it was Endometriosis. After surgery and returning home, we followed up with my OB/GYN and found out the only way to determine what the spots were would to be another surgery.

Finally on May 21st, 2020, three days before my 17th birthday we were able to have my ablation surgery. It was confirmed endometriosis on both my right and left ovarian tubes which were burned off, this created a world with which I was unfamiliar. We immediately changed my birth control to the IUD which stopped my period however it didn't stop my pain. We began adding more medications to try to slow the progression of my endometriosis growth. Nothing helped or relieved pain including high painkillers that I feared would be addictive as a growing teen.

Before long, the pain became unbearable again causing me to go under the knife for another ablation surgery on September 4th, 2021, finding it again along my right and left ovarian tubes and the walls surrounding my uterus. This was my senior year of high school. The COVID-19 pandemic had taken away my senior year and here we were creating a bigger mess and making me more susceptible to contracting COVID. But I graduated and I thought wow here is where I can make a difference. I left home and began my years at the University of Alabama, where I started advocating on campus to raise awareness for endometriosis. I was featured in my campus' women and gender sources center hotspot email!

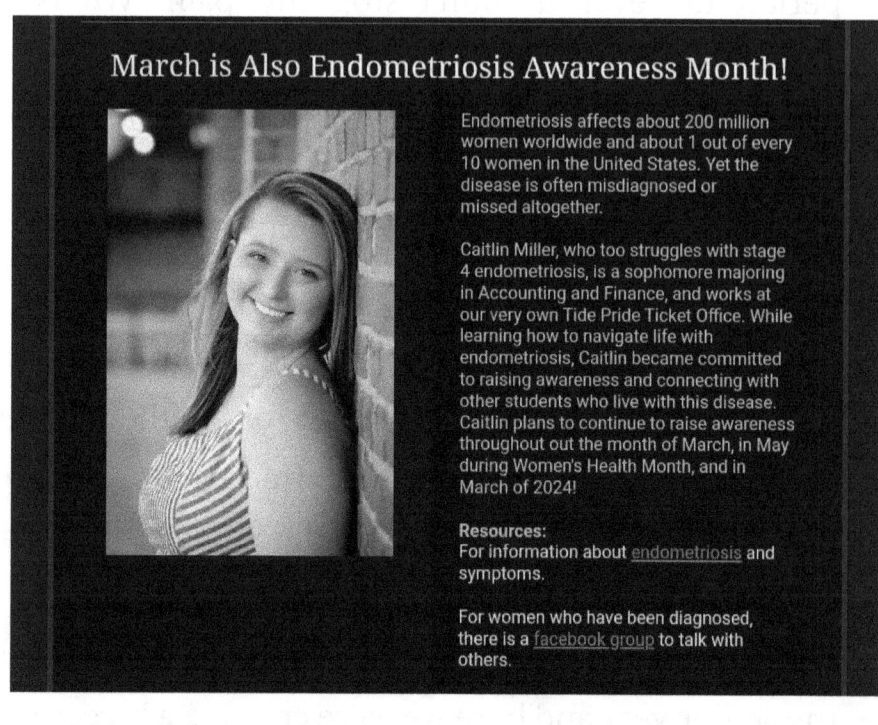

### March is Also Endometriosis Awareness Month!

Endometriosis affects about 200 million women worldwide and about 1 out of every 10 women in the United States. Yet the disease is often misdiagnosed or missed altogether.

Caitlin Miller, who too struggles with stage 4 endometriosis, is a sophomore majoring in Accounting and Finance, and works at our very own Tide Pride Ticket Office. While learning how to navigate life with endometriosis, Caitlin became committed to raising awareness and connecting with other students who live with this disease. Caitlin plans to continue to raise awareness throughout out the month of March, in May during Women's Health Month, and in March of 2024!

**Resources:**
For information about endometriosis and symptoms.

For women who have been diagnosed, there is a facebook group to talk with others.

As my freshman year began the pain started getting worse, I began missing classes until March 29th, 2022. During a math exam, I began having pains just like in 2019. I felt I had to use the restroom and then I felt nauseous. How could this be, I changed my diet as much as a broke college kid could; I was walking everywhere to increase physical activity, why me? I immediately ran into the restroom and called my mom. I explained everything and immediately she began calling friends to get me to the hospital, all my friends were in class due to exams. Surely my mom took a step far worse than calling for an ambulance, she called my ex-boyfriend. He ran into the math and science building, pulling me out of the bathroom with his new girlfriend and rushing me to the emergency room. Man, talk about pain and embarrassment.

I was kept overnight for pain management, where both my mom and new boyfriend rushed to be by my side as soon as possible. The ER doctor told me to follow up with my OB/GYN, which I did, and he prescribed me Lupron Depot®. I did not want to throw myself into menopause, the thought of never being able to be a mom scared me. Being away from family at college was already hard enough, and with my history of depression my mother and I decided it was best not to even begin to take the drug.

After this my teachers began asking me about my absences and that is when I met a co-worker of my professor who told me about *Nancys Nook* a Facebook group for women with endometriosis. I began talking to her about her friend who had been through it, and she told me about a specialist in Tennessee, Robert Furr an endometriosis specialist, who her friend had been to and had not had pain in three years.

This was my chance; I immediately called my mom and told her everything. We immediately researched him and began looking at getting an appointment with him while she began gathering all my medical documentation. Finally, we were able to schedule my first appointment with him. I explained to him after he read over my history that it felt like my doctor had given up and just wanted to shut down everything in my reproductive area. He explained that ablation surgery just burned off the tip of the endo and does not fully remove it whereas excision is taking a tool and cutting all the way to the root of it and removing it.

I thought possibly this could be what makes me a "normal" teen. He explained, however; there was no cure for endo and that this would be a lifelong battle. I explained that I knew the statistics of infertility in women with endo is roughly 50%, and that when I graduate college I want to try for children. He explained that is a common worry with all women he sees around my age up to 10 years older than me.

We scheduled surgery after discussing with my mom that we do not have many options left. On April 14th, 2022, we had my surgery where he said he found it EVERYWHERE. It was noted in my file to be on both ovarian tubes, behind my ovaries, along my walls, on my bladder and even on my anus. For months I felt a great deal of relief but roughly 10 months later I began to feel extreme amounts of pain and began bleeding.

I was out of school for spring break and decided to just pop into my original OB/GYN to make sure everything was okay. He immediately told me he refused to do another surgery on me and prescribed me Letrozole® which would once again shut down my reproductive system. I immediately contacted my specialist who sent me nonaddictive pain meds to help me until I could get into the office to see him. He has already scheduled a "Second Look" surgery to remove any new growth and I will be undergoing my 5th surgery for endo on July 12th, 2023, as a 20-year-old.

---

Again, we see with Caitlin's story the likewise affects endometriosis has on her. We once again see a young lady who struggled as a young girl just starting her period into adulthood with this horrible debilitating disease. Experts estimate that more than 11% of females aged 15–44 in the United States have endometriosis (Mph, 2022).[4]

---

[4] Mph, Z. S. (2022, January 21). What to know about endometriosis in teenagers. https://www.medicalnewstoday.com/articles/endometriosis-in-teens

# 6

## KERRY ELLIOT

Back when I was 13, I knew in myself that my body was not right; to suffer in pain every day. I would have crippling migraines and severe cramping, and like a stabbing pain right around my stomach and groin area, also causing me to be violently sick. When telling the doctor this, I always got fobbed off with, "It's just IBS." I knew, this was not right, about any of those things.

Around ten years later my mum was having a brain operation, however; I spoke to her neurologist and explained that I had been going to the doctor for the exact same symptoms as my mum! Within five minutes he had me going for an MRI scan and revealed that I had a 'Chiari Malformation' which is pressure on the brain. This causes me migraines and headaches everyday along with fainting, and there is no cure. If it were not for him listening to me, I never would have been diagnosed.

Years gone by suffering with the same pains in my stomach, I would go to A&E a lot, because all I could describe the pain is like being carved out like a pumpkin, or feeling like I had a chronic hangover headache. Sometimes I would think I was dying. Whilst at A&E, they could never find out what it was. They always thought it was to do with my appendix or ovaries and sent me away with Tramadol® each time.

I struggled a lot with being unwell, praying each night that I would wake up and be normal and have a normal health, but that never came around. I was exhausted visiting three different hospitals and doctor appointments and just receiving bad news after bad news or no plan forward.

I would be sick on a regular basis, hanging over the toilet at all hours of the morning, and when it came to 'that time' of the month, I was bed bound for a week. Straight feeling like I was repeatedly having a kick in. One night in A&E, I was sick as a dog and in complete pain when the doctor said. "When did you have your laparoscopy?" Which I replied, "What do you mean?" feeling totally baffled.

The doctor showed me the letter from the hospital that was from the beginning of 2017 stating that I should have been going for a laparoscopy for endometriosis.

> "Endometriosis (en-doe-me-tree-O-sis) is an often-painful disorder in which tissue similar to the tissue that normally lines the inside of the uterus – the endometrium – grows outside of your uterus. Endometriosis most commonly involves the ovaries, fallopian tubes, and the tissue lining your pelvis."

This chronic illness can also cause infertility and leaves your body most days feeling and looking like your nine months pregnant. Now the anger built up inside me because I had been walking into a brick wall for around 12 years for my own GP to not pass on this information and it was now going into 2019.

When I was able to move whilst filled with pain killers, I went around to the GP and demanded that operation. Few months later, I was at St. John's going for a laparoscopic surgery. I was not allowed my parents inside with me or when I woke up from the operation which was very daunting and scary going through it all alone.

There were complications during the operation and some of my endometriosis had turned 'old' and was sticking to my kidneys and tubes so they could only laser some away as I would die if they had to cut the old endo away. Soon as I came out of high dependence, I fainted 7 times in the space of an hour. The recovery was terrible, I could not bend or walk, and my stitches took forever to heal properly.

The pain lightened for a couple of months but has all grew back again and is back in style. Being crippled in bed, not being able to drink alcohol as it attacks my body, cannot eat takeaways, or drink any fizzy juice or just any day-to-day life experiences without feeling like I need to sit or lie down. I lie in bed begging for it to stop. Taking Tramadol® and other strong painkillers does not even take the edge off. The heartburn and sickness feel like it is never going to stop.

To say it is difficult to live with a debilitating, chronic condition is the very least. Having the incapacitating symptoms, being misdiagnosed, and speaking to professionals who quite obviously do not understand it and not having certain hopes in my future has made it unpredictable and all that more difficult. Then there are the challenges like needing to speak about this "taboo" subject, dealing with closed minded people or those who feel you are exaggerating, forceful opinions, and false information being spread, lack of understanding, and there is so much more.

I also got diagnosed with 'POTS,' which is, "Postural Tachycardia Syndrome (PoTS) is an abnormal increase in heart rate that occurs after sitting up or standing. Some typical symptoms include dizziness and fainting. It is sometimes known as Postural Orthostatic Tachycardia Syndrome."

I have collapsed a couple times in public places; I always feel a rush of heat throughout my body followed by vomiting and then collapsing. My heart rate usually can sit at 148BPM just sitting, and the hospital will not let me drive it is too dangerous. Through all of this, I still try and work as a team leader in a private nursery. So, working hours and am terribly busy, Which I have been doing for ten years.

I had to give up most things I like to do or would like to do in the future as my body cannot handle being in overly busy places or staying outside for overly prolonged periods of time. I carry around different pills in my bag and always need to plan ahead in case I collapse, or I am sick or take dizzy turns. I also have been battling these chronic illnesses with no cure for 13 years, which ended up leading me to take antidepressants which is the only thing that keeps me sane.

Never take your health for granted as there are many people begging and wishing they could wake up and just feel okay and not have every day as a battle just to move around and function. If you know your body and know something is not right, keep persevering and pushing the doctor to listen. It has taken me years and years for just one doctor to finally listen to me. I know you can feel like you are in a dark hole, and no one is listening, understanding, or helping, but keep going.

I would never wish these conditions on my worst enemy and some days you think 'What's the point in life being crippled and majorly suffering in pain every day.'. Thankfully, everyone who knows me knows I go above and beyond for people and always try to have people smiling and staying positive. I am thankful for everyone who has stuck by me, and my family are there for me every day. Keeping me positive and to keep fighting it all. One day I pray for a cure for all conditions as no one can see the excruciating level of pain that your body is suffering and because you put a brave face on, and we put on a brave face making people think, "it cannot be that sore.".

Kerry is from Scottland. I found it particularly interesting how even in other countries they experience the same lack of knowledge and understanding surrounding endometriosis. What I originally thought may be just an American problem, clearly was a worldwide dilemma. Provided, countries overseas provide better care than here in the United States in most cases; the need for awareness and knowledge very clearly is needed in all corners of the world. We hope this book can help provide a better understanding to everyone who reads it.

# 7

## MELISSA IRWIN

My older sister and I have always struggled with heavy, painful periods. My mom always struggled with them too and told us it was normal, so I never gave it much thought.

*"It's just what women have to deal with. Take some Ibuprofen and you'll be fine."*, my mom would say.

This would later be something I would be told by health professionals all too often. Was being in excruciating pain normal? Ok I guess they are the professionals and know what they are talking about... Right?

2006. The first time I had pain during sex, I was 19 years old and was staying at a hotel with my then boyfriend. It felt like an explosion in my lower abdominal area, and I immediately doubled over into the fetal position. I laid there for God knows how long, my boyfriend beside himself not knowing what to do. He wasn't much help, but I don't know what he even could have done for me anyway.

I remember I thought taking a hot bath might help, but it didn't. Nothing did, so I went to the ER, and they sent me home with some Ibuprofen and said to rest. No tests, no scans, nothing. I felt like I was making a big deal out of nothing.

"It's just what women have to deal with, right?", I thought to myself. My boyfriend thought that I was exaggerating too, since that's what the doctors were basically saying.

2007. Things started escalating with my boyfriend. Anytime I would say sex hurt he would act like I was inconveniencing him, like I was just trying to ruin it somehow. It got to the point that if it hurt, he ignored me and kept going. I was young and didn't have the best example to know how to stand up for myself. I know I should have kicked him to the curb long before things got to this point, but I thought I loved him. After a while, I thought I was pregnant, so we sat my parents down and told them. My parents are Christian and don't believe in sex before marriage. They highly encouraged us to get married. Since we were staying at their house, I felt a lot of pressure from them to say yes.

A few weeks passed and I had a breakdown. At this time, I had long hair that went almost to my thighs. I woke up in the middle of the night, having a lot of abdominal pain, and my hair was wrapped around my face and neck. I got up, went to the bathroom, and started crying. I grabbed my mom's scissors and started chopping off my hair. I started feeling better, but I looked into the mirror and started bawling my eyes out.

I fell to the floor and curled into a ball. My dad heard me and came in to check on me. He saw me and smiled a knowing smile. He scoops me up and just holds me while I wail. He told me everything will be ok and that he is there.

"Your hair will grow back, sweety-pie", he says to me. "Daddy, I think I lost the baby!" I cry out. "I know, little-one. It's ok, your mother and I are here for you." He said, while rocking me, and stroking my freshly chopped hair. I just melted into his arms and sobbed for a long time.

The next morning my mom evened out my hair into a cute bob. She didn't shame me for cutting my long hair that she loved so much. She knew it was not what was important at that time. I didn't see a doctor because I had no insurance and could not pay for it, so it went undiagnosed, but I knew what happened.

Eventually my boyfriend cheated on me, and I found out from a mutual friend what he was doing. The relationship ended, but my pain did not. He left me with a lot of damage, both physical and emotional.

Anytime I had pain, I would just take Ibuprofen and just ride it out. I worked full time as a manager at a fast-food chain, so I just did my best to ignore it and carry on.

*"It's just what women have to deal with"* ...

This would be my life for another year until I met the man I would eventually marry. He never hurt me. He was gentle and understanding when I told him something hurt. Sex wasn't important to him, he just wanted to be around me. Sex was just a bonus. With him, my feelings mattered. My words mattered. We went a bit fast, and we were engaged within 7 months of dating. We just knew we wanted to spend the rest of our lives together.

2009. Fast forward to our wedding night. The first time we were intimate as a married couple, I had another "explosion" in my lower abdominal area. My husband immediately carried me to the car and drove me to the ER. When we got there, we didn't have to wait long before being seen by the sweetest doctor I have ever met. I told him that my sister had been diagnosed with PCOS, and we suspected I might have the same thing.

We have similar symptoms, but I had more attacks than she did. He took this very seriously and wanted me to have a transvaginal ultrasound, the only problem being that there was no technician there at midnight. He called in the technician to do the ultrasound. When she got there, she looked like she had just woken up and was not happy. She wheeled me to the radiology department and instructed me to lie down. I do so and she inserts the probe. She is not gentle. She is irritated and did not take me seriously. I cry out in pain, and she ignores me.

She finds 14 cysts on my left ovary, signs of a ruptured cyst also on my left ovary, and free fluid in the cul-de-sac. They do not find my right ovary. The doctor told me that his daughter has the same condition and that as much as he feels for me, there is not much he can do. He gives me some Vicodin and sends me home. This would be the last time I go to the ER for this. As sweet as he was, there was no point. They would just send me home with pain meds, and I can do that at home and not feel like an inconvenience.

> *"It's just what women have to deal with. Take some Ibuprofen and you'll be fine."*, my mother's words forever in the back of my mind.

For a while I'm able to get government insurance so I can see a women's health doctor. She is nice enough and says that I probably do have PCOS but does not do any testing or scans of any kind. I didn't know any better and trusted her judgment.

2012. I think I am pregnant again. Every test I take comes back negative, so I went to see my doctor and the test comes back negative. I have every tell-tail sign of pregnancy and my doctor tells me that it's common with PCOS. After a month and a half, I still have not gotten my period and the tests are still coming back negative. I just started doing things like I am pregnant though, just in case. After about 2 months, my belly started growing, but tests are still negative. My mom tells me that it is possible to have a false negative and that I probably am pregnant. I was really excited, and my husband was too. We were on our way to start a family, something I have wanted my whole life.

Then one day, I started bleeding heavily and had terrible lower abdominal pain. I called my doctor's office, and the nurse told me to come in right away. When I got there, they led me to her office, and I waited for the doctor. When she comes in, she is visibly irritated and says,

*"You are not pregnant; you are just having a bad period. This happens with PCOS."* and walks out of the room.

She did not do a physical examination or any tests. I go home, my husband is at work, so I just cry in my bed for hours. All the while I'm bleeding heavily, and it is super clumpy. I knew there was something different about this. This was not just a "bad period". There was no other doctor I could see for a second opinion; she was the only gynecologist in the area that my insurance would pay for. I took an ibuprofen and hoped that I would be fine.

***"You're going to have to come to terms with the fact that this is probably all in your head."*** She said to me once.

I went back to her, and she put me on birth control. She said it would manage my symptoms. I started taking it and it made me feel extremely depressed and suicidal. I couldn't handle it, so I stopped taking them. My doctor told me that all of them would make me feel that way and it was my only option. I did not take the birth control again and she just looked at me funny like I just wanted attention. I in fact did not want this attention. I just wanted to be normal.

I was really embarrassed... I stopped going in to see her except for my yearly pap smears. There was still no other doctor II could see in my area that would take my insurance. I thought I was crazy and didn't want to bother anyone else with the pain that must be "all in my head".

I went into a deep depression. I lost my insurance because my husband and I both had jobs, but couldn't afford the insurance our employers offered, and we made too much to qualify for government assistance. I went to work but didn't want to go anywhere or see anyone. I stopped wanting intimacy from my husband and we started growing apart. He understood, but I pushed him away. Hard. It wasn't only because of the pain; I had given up on life. I wasn't going to be a mother, and that killed me inside. That was what I wanted more than anything else.

2016. Years go on like a blur and my husband and I both grow more and more depressed. I start to have vision problems and end up having to quit my job because I can't see anymore. Again, no insurance and no money to pay to see a doctor. Even after I quit, my husband still made too much money to qualify for assistance. A few months passed and my husband started having medical issues himself and went on medical leave and was eventually laid off.

We were able to get government assistance again and I was able to go to the eye doctor. I had hereditary cataracts and was able to get surgery to get lens implants. I didn't try to speak to anyone about my abdominal pain. It was manageable with pain meds, and it wasn't the most pressing matter to me at the time. I didn't want to waste my time just for a doctor to tell me it's all in my head.

2017. I found it harder and harder to cope with the pain through pain meds alone. I decided to try my luck with a new doctor. A new clinic had just opened that would take my insurance. The doctor I met was kind and listened to what I was telling her. She was mortified when I told her how my previous doctor brushed me off. She told me she thought it was Endometriosis. I had never heard of it before, and she explained it to me. It made a lot of sense and would explain a lot of my symptoms. She sent in an order for an ultrasound and referred me to a specialist. The "specialist" she referred me to is at the same clinic I had gone to previously. I got scared and did not go. I didn't trust them. I continued to manage my pain with pain meds. I switched from Ibuprofen to Naproxen. This seemed to help a bit more.

2021. I started having pain with urination and bowel movements. The first time this happened I thought I would never be able to poop again. I couldn't bring myself to let it happen, it hurt so much. Finally, I just had to let it hurt. I screamed on the toilet for about 20 minutes while I tried to relieve myself. I made another appointment with the doctor. I explained to her that I did not want to go back to that clinic. She referred me to a specialist one town over.

I went to my appointment this time and told him everything that was going on. When I was explaining the type of pain I had during sex, he was visibly uncomfortable and chuckled at me. This was supposed to be a professional and this was very serious to me. He did an examination and ultrasound in his office and found a 3.5 cm cyst on my left ovary. That was all he was concerned about. He told me to come back in 3 months to see if it has changed in size. I went back to my GP and explained what happened and that I wanted to see someone else. She referred me to someone else in the same clinic.

2022. My first appointment she got called away to deliver a baby so another doctor from the city was filling in for her. He did an examination and ultrasound. This doctor took a broader look at what was going on instead of just focusing on my ovary. He saw that I have "kissing ovaries". They had fallen to the bottom of my abdominal cavity and my uterus was tilted toward my colon. This was a tell-tail sign of Endometriosis. They could no longer ignore me. I had a follow up appointment with the doctor I was supposed to see, and she referred me to UCSF. Finally, I would be getting some answers.

2023. In July Dr. Traci Ito at UCSF performed laparoscopic surgery and took two 4cm cysts (endometriomas) off of my left ovary. They did some exploring and ended up having to take my entire right ovary (the one they could never find) and fallopian tube. The ovary was covered in endometrial tissue and was fused to my uterus. In the report they sent me it said that it exploded after they took it out. That very well could have happened inside of me.

In conclusion, I have read many articles about why it takes women so long to receive treatment. Most of them talk about how women don't accurately gauge their pain and let their doctor know. This is entirely inaccurate. Most women get dismissed and told they are overreacting or that it's all in their head. Awareness needs to be brought to the fact that, especially in small towns, doctors don't really care or know much about

Endometriosis, and women across the globe suffer for way longer than they should because of it.

# 8

## STACEY SMITH

From the age of 13 years old, I suffered with very heavy and extremely painful periods. On many occasions, I was not able to go to school and had to stay in bed.

I had numerous GP appointments but was told the pain was normal and was prescribed PONSTAN® which is for mild period pains. When I was 17 years old, I realized what I was experiencing was not normal - I began having severe labour-like pains and hot and cold sweats. I sometimes passed out, vomited and at times had to crawl around on the floor just to get around as the pain was so severe.

The abdominal pain could come on very suddenly. My stomach was swollen which made me look pregnant - I found this very embarrassing and distressing. Others would make comments and ask how far along my pregnancy was. I was aged 15 (a virgin). Friends had to phone my dad to ask him to come in the car to collect me. I actually thought I was going to die. I continued to go to my GP, but the only suggestion was to start taking the contraceptive pill which I was told would help with the extreme pain, bloating and heavy bleeding but it never did.

I tried everything, hormonal and non-hormonal treatments, but nothing worked – in fact they made the bleeding worse. I was checked regularly for Sexually Transmitted Infections and Sexually Transmitted Diseases – the tests were always negative. I had numerous pregnancy tests as medical staff considered I could be miscarrying – I knew this was never the case.

I was persuaded to have a contraceptive implant (a rod implanted under the skin of my upper arm) as I was told this would certainly help. It didn't, I bled constantly for the 3 months I had it. I wanted it removed, but staff refused until I said that if they did not remove it, I would rip it out myself.

For the next 4 years, I tried to get a referral to a gynecologist so I could be properly investigated – I had never had any proper investigations (only a number of internal examinations and I was always told everything was fine). It was a constant battle and a fight to get anyone to listen.

When I was 22 years old, I had my first gynecology appointment and it was agreed to carry out some investigations – a transvaginal ultrasound scan, a hysteroscopy, hysterosalpingogram – none of which showed anything except a heart-shaped bicornuate uterus. It was then agreed to carry out a laparoscopy which found widespread adhesions and fibroids.

I asked why the adhesions and fibroids had not been removed during the laparoscopy and was told that they would not cause my severe symptoms and it was better to leave them alone. I was furious and for the next 2 years fought to have them removed.

When I was 24 years old, I had another laparoscopy to remove the fibroids and adhesions. After the surgery I was told that I had widespread, deeply infiltrative endometriosis. I didn't know what endometriosis was and I was told it was nothing to worry about. I asked if endometriosis should be there and I was told no. I became agitated and asked why it had not been removed - I also felt that if the fibroids and adhesions had been removed 2 years before, the endometriosis would have been found then.

Medical staff said the equipment necessary to remove endometriosis was not available in that hospital but that I could have it done privately. It's always about money – I could hardly keep a job because of the effects of endometriosis.

What I didn't know then was that endometriosis could be treated and removed by laparoscopy – the surgery I had just had.

I was prescribed Decapeptyl® injections but was not told that although this induced a chemical menopause, I still needed to use contraception as it was still possible to become pregnant. If I became pregnant there was a risk that the baby would be born with no limbs. Also, I was not prescribed hormone replacement therapy while having Decapeptyl® injections to prevent horrific side effects – mood swings, hot flashes, night sweats etc. It was only when I experienced these side effects and did some online research that I discovered this. Without HRT Decapeptyl® had a terrible effect on me – I felt I was going mad. I was like a woman possessed, angry, argumentative, making others cry – this was totally out of character for me. I understand Decapeptyl® remains in your system for 6 months and when I stopped the injections, I suffered panic attacks and felt as though I was having a heart attack (rapid heart rate and palpitations). Thankfully despite not using contraception, I did not become pregnant.

By the time I was 26 years old I was still trying to have the endometriosis removed but doctors were still refusing to do this. I was referred for IVF despite the fact it was unlikely to be successful due to extent of the endometriosis. I was set up to fail, I was struggling physically, mentally, socially and by this point I had no career or friends. I now had anger issues, depression, and worsening endometriosis – it was destroying my life. I now experienced severe pain on an almost daily basis.

Between the ages of 26 and 27 years old, I had IVF treatment. I was told to give up smoking but got no help with this. The first IVF procedure had to be postponed as I developed a clot in my womb. In preparation for IVF, I had to give myself injections to decrease my egg production (apparently, I produce too many eggs). Of the 6 eggs that were harvested, only 4 were viable and only 2 actually were fertilized.

However, I received a phone call to say that neither of the 2 fertilized eggs had made it past stage 3 and it was highly unlikely they would progress further overnight. I was asked, very insensitively, whether I wanted them to be discarded into the bin or kept overnight. Although I was assured nothing would change overnight, I said I wanted to wait. I was called the next day and told there had been no change, so they were discarded into the bin as if they were nothing. I immediately started smoking again and my depression worsened - I felt hopeless.

Now I understand that even if my eggs had been implanted into me, it would have been pointless as endometriosis affects egg quality, prevents implantation, and even if it does implant it may not make it very far on anyway as endometriosis is a hostile environment. This whole process was pointless and affected me very badly emotionally and mentally – the professionals involved knew it was not going to work so why would they put anyone through this?

The IVF team were keen to discuss a 2nd attempt however because of my declining mental health I did not want this. I felt I could barely look after myself, therefore what good would I be to a child, so I refused. I was in so much pain – everywhere – spine, pelvis, stomach, anus, vagina, ovaries, thighs, and legs- I was at the point where I could no longer function. I spent most of the time in bed crying, screaming, swearing– I used hot water bottles, took scalding hot baths, electric heat pads, heat sprays, freeze sprays, but nothing helped. I could not look after my home either. My life had broken down in every way – I felt inadequate as I could not have children.

This affected me more when I was with others who could have children; baby scan, conversations about fertility and motherhood were unpleasant. I couldn't tell what my mood was going to be like from one day to the next and I would eventually after keeping quiet about my feelings for so long start to express them no matter what or to who. I was considered rude, but I'm not actually rude, I was just being truthful. I had experienced years of not being respected or treated sensitively so I responded in the very same way towards others.

I continued to be very angry about the neglect I had suffered from medical professionals and the permanent damage the endometriosis has caused me physically. I decided to go along to my local endometriosis support group, but I only went a few times - I was the only person there who did not have children.

Additionally, most other members, unlike me, had undergone surgery to remove endometriosis (and they did not seem to have had any problems getting this done). I realized these support groups were not for everyone and definitely not for me – in fact I received some derogatory comments despite other members knowing my situation.

I did however get some useful information for example how to get a referral to another health board to see specialists. I spoke to my GP who referred me to a specialist, and I waited in the hope that I would get the help and treatment I needed.

In November 2016 at the age of 28 I had ureteric stents inserted in preparation for a laparoscopy. After the surgery, I initially felt fine, however I started to suffer excruciating pain - I was not given any pain relief and as no infection or other reason could be found for the cause of the pain, I was sent home. (I vomited constantly during the journey home) I was told that there would be blood in my urine for a few days, but this continued for months. The constant pain also continued, and I was very lethargic.

I was due to have the laparoscopy in December 2016, however, my period started, and I had been told that if I had my period, the laparoscopy would not be done. However, due to the length of time I had waited a decision was made to go ahead with the surgery. I was also told also they had found signs of infection the source of which was the ureteric stents.

I had the 1st laparoscopy in December 2015 and despite being told that if any endometriosis was found it would be removed, it was not. I was told the disease was so bad it required a team of specialists to carry out the surgery. I was very angry and once again felt I had been neglected and badly let down by medical professionals. So, the 2nd laparoscopy was done December 2016, but I had to have stents inserted beforehand in November 2016.

Immediately following the surgery December 2016, I actually felt the best I had felt all my life, but I now know it was only the effect of the morphine. As I felt so good, I asked to go home but they were reluctant and advised I stay at least 3 days. I felt fine - I insisted they remove the catheter and everything else and to get me a discharge sheet. (I had forgotten all about the prior infection and that I had not been given any antibiotics) I was just exhilarated that for once I did not feel horrific pain. I was discharged home that night and I still felt great the following day. However, the day after that I experienced horrific pain which went on for months.

I lost weight, drifted in and out of consciousness, was unable to get up and barely able to eat. My family contacted the doctor numerous times and finally the doctor came out to see me and prescribed morphine. He told my family they had difficulty inserting even the smallest stent and it had not been possible to get one in – I would later find out this was not the case - both were in and had to be "rammed in".
In March 2017, I received phone messages from my GP asking me to attend the surgery immediately, but after 5 months of trying to persuade them that something was wrong, I was actually beginning to feel better so did not want to waste my time. I did go to the surgery though, and staff took my blood pressure and immediately called an ambulance as they considered I was going to have a heart attack.

They took me to hospital where I was weighed, and I was asked if I was anorexic as I was under 6 stone in weight. I had various investigations including a CT scan of the abdomen with pelvis contrast. The tests showed that I was hypotensive, pyrexial and tachycardic, I had pyelonephritis, hydronephrosis (despite inserted stents), sepsis and I was hypothermic. I had to have regular injections to stop blood clots forming to prevent the need for amputation, regular intravenous fluids, and intravenous antibiotics as well as regular ECGs and blood pressure checks. I remained in hospital for a week and was told I was one day away from death.

I was discharged home on antibiotics and was referred to a dietician for supplement drinks (it was actually over a year until I was seen by a dietician). I suffered with insomnia and had extreme kidney pain, urinary urgency, and stress incontinence.

The urinary problems only started after the stents were inserted and I believed they would be resolved when they were removed. In April 2017 at the age of 29 years the stents were finally removed, but nothing changed. I have been prescribed antibiotics on a long-term basis to prevent recurring kidney infections and to prevent sepsis.

Meanwhile, my endometriosis remained but my appointments with specialists were all cancelled with no explanation. I had to attend my GP regularly to ask to be re-referred to the specialists. I was and remain very concerned about the lack of monitoring of my kidney function.

Finally, in 2018, I was given an appointment which was not cancelled and at this appointment, it was agreed that I would be put on a 12-week waiting list for a laparotomy -I was told it would be a much larger incision so the specialist would be able to get a better look inside to understand the full extent of the disease.

I was also given laparotomy information sheets explaining why I was having this surgery rather than a laparoscopy procedure. Shortly after this I received a letter stating I had exceeded the waiting list times and to call them. I did and they explained I would have to wait another year but would definitely have the surgery in the summer of 2019. I did not have surgery in 2019 and then in March 2020, the country went into lockdown because of the Covid-19 pandemic. I called again to be told I would definitely have surgery in the summer of 2020.

In 2021- my GP wrote again but still no date for surgery. In December 2022, I got a call from the hospital to let me know there was a date for surgery – a laparoscopy.

However, this was not the surgery I was waiting for – I was to have a laparotomy. In January 2023, I received another phone call from the hospital letting me know I was at the top of the waiting list and a telephone appointment had been made for me to speak to a gynecologist. I questioned the reason for the telephone appointment and once again questioned the surgery I was to undergo. I asked that the telephone appointment with a gynecologist be cancelled.

I submitted a complaint and a request for a copy of my medical files. During a phone consultation with the consultant, he denied he had ever said I was to have a laparotomy despite the fact that someone was with me during the appointment.

When I did receive a copy of my notes, much of the information was redacted, however, I had a copy of my medical notes from some years before with no redactions and the information was there. My notes had been doctored – for example they said I had been prescribed antibiotics – I wasn't, they said I refused surgery in 2018 – I did not, they said the date I was put on waiting list was 2021 – it was actually 2018. I do not want another laparoscopy as the one I had in 2016 did not relieve my pain.

The consultant has suggested I transfer to another health board as there is no trust left between me and the team. Moving to the Greater Glasgow and Clyde Health Board is not an option as it would mean 4 hours of travelling which I cannot tolerate due to pain and nausea not to mention the cost of fuel. Following my complaint, they advised I could contact the SPSO. I was offered a laparoscopy on the 25th of February 2023 which I had to refuse due to personal reasons.

I underwent a laparoscopy on the 15th of March 2023 to remove widespread Endometriosis again. It was also noted my womb was weak (did not find this out till report was sent out month or so later) I was supposed to receive a call the week later for follow up but the week after no call came.

"Endometriosis – A legacy no Auntie wants to leave her nieces".

Endometriosis is negatively life impacting – Endometriosis has caused me:
- Impact on education, career, and finances
- To lose / breakdown of friendships /
- relationships (Due to infertility stuck while others move, pain and, social impact)
- Depression
- Self-isolation and loneliness (no one understands)
- Agoraphobia
- Affects mentally, physically, socially, and emotionally.
- Infertility and psychological impacts
- Long term anger issues (medical neglect, gas lighting, insensitivities towards infertility)

# PART 2

## INFERTILITY AND LOSS

# 9

# ENDOMETRIOSIS AND INFERTILITY

Infertility is one of the most significant impacts of endometriosis. It is estimated that around 30-50% of women with endometriosis experience infertility. The exact mechanisms behind this association are not fully understood, but there are several theories:

Distorted Pelvic Anatomy: The presence of endometrial implants can lead to distorted pelvic anatomy, altering the normal structure and function of the reproductive organs. This can result in decreased egg quality, impaired hormone production, and decreased sperm motility, all of which contribute to infertility.

b) Inflammation and Scar Tissue: Endometriosis causes inflammation and the formation of scar tissue. This can affect the ovaries, fallopian tubes, and the delicate structures involved in fertility. Consequently, the fallopian tubes may become blocked, preventing the egg from reaching the uterus and the sperm from reaching the egg.

c) Immune Dysfunction: Some evidence suggests that endometriosis may trigger immune dysfunction, leading to an abnormal immunological response that impacts fertility. Altered immune responses can compromise the chances of successful implantation and the maintenance of a healthy pregnancy.

Assisted Reproductive Technologies (ART) and Endometriosis:
For women who experience infertility due to endometriosis, various assisted reproductive technologies (ART) can be used to improve the chances of conception. These may include in vitro fertilization

(IVF), intrauterine insemination (IUI), and other procedures.

IVF is often the most effective treatment option for women with severe endometriosis. It involves stimulating the ovaries to produce multiple eggs, retrieving the eggs, fertilizing them in a laboratory, and transferring the resulting embryos back to the uterus. However, the success rates for IVF vary based on individual factors such as age, disease severity, and the presence of other fertility issues.

Risk of Stillbirths:
Recent studies have indicated a potential link between endometriosis and an increased risk of stillbirths. A 2020 study published in the journal Human Reproduction reported that women with endometriosis had a higher risk of stillbirth compared to those without the condition. The specific reasons behind this relationship are still being investigated, but it is believed that the chronic inflammation associated with endometriosis may play a role.

Managing Endometriosis and Improving Fertility Outcomes:

Effective management of endometriosis can help improve fertility outcomes and reduce the risk of stillbirth. Treatment options include:

Pain management: Medications such as nonsteroidal anti-inflammatory drugs (NSAIDs) and hormonal therapies can help alleviate pain associated with endometriosis.

Surgery: Depending on the severity and location of endometriotic lesions, surgery may be recommended. Laparoscopic excision or ablation of endometriosis can restore pelvic anatomy, reduce inflammation, and enhance fertility outcomes.

Fertility treatments: ART, as mentioned earlier, can be used to help women with endometriosis achieve pregnancy. Consulting with a reproductive endocrinologist can provide personalized advice based on individual circumstances.

Psychological Well-being and Support:
It is crucial to acknowledge the emotional toll that endometriosis, infertility, and stillbirths can have on individuals and couples. The psychological impact of these conditions should not be underestimated, and seeking appropriate support, such as counseling or support groups, can be beneficial.

Endometriosis significantly impacts fertility, leading to an increased risk of infertility and possibly stillbirths. While there is ongoing research in this field, a multidisciplinary approach involving healthcare professionals from various specialties is important to address the medical and psychological aspects of these conditions. Continued research efforts aim to better understand the mechanisms behind endometriosis-related infertility and find effective treatment options for affected individuals.

[5]

---

[5] 1. American Society for Reproductive Medicine. (2019). Endometriosis: A guide for patients. Retrieved from https://www.asrm.org/globalassets/asrm/asrm-content/news-and-publications/practice-guidelines/released/your-guide-to-endometriosis.pdf

2. Johnson, N. P., & Hummelshoj, L. (2013). Consensus on current management of endometriosis. Human Reproduction, 28(6), 1552-1568.

3. Vercellini, P., et al. (2014). Medical treatment of endometriosis-associated recurrent pregnancy loss: A systematic review and meta-analysis. Human Reproduction Update, 20(4), 493-515.

4. Nnoaham, K. E., et al. (2012). Impact of endometriosis on quality of life and work productivity: a multicenter study across ten countries. Fertility and Sterility, 96(2), 366-373.

5. Stephansson, O., et al. (2020). Endometriosis and stillbirth: A nationwide cohort registry study. Human Reproduction, 35(9), 2171-2177.

# 10

## IMPACT OF ENDOMETRIOSIS AND INFERTILITY

You do everything right. You eat healthy, exercise, limit stress, and take your prenatal vitamins. You've been trying to conceive for over a year and finally see those two pink lines on the pregnancy test. Excitement and joy flood through you at the thought of holding your baby in just a few short months. But then the bleeding starts. And the cramps. You rush to the doctor, hoping and praying it's nothing serious. But the ultrasound confirms your worst fear: there is no heartbeat. Your world comes crashing down in an instant. The painful reality of another loss sinks in as you struggle to understand why this keeps happening. You feel broken and defeated, wondering if you'll ever become a mother.

For women battling endometriosis, the road to motherhood is often lined with heartbreak and loss. Despite doing everything in your power to achieve a healthy pregnancy, your body continues to fail you for reasons outside of your control. Each month you hope this will be the one, only to face disappointment again. The pain of endometriosis is difficult enough but coupled with the anguish of infertility and infant loss, it becomes unbearable. This is a story of one woman's journey through the deepest despair to find hope on the other side. My story. Your story. The story of all women who refuse to give up hope in the face of unimaginable odds.

**Understanding Endometriosis and Its Impact on Fertility**

Endometriosis occurs when tissue similar to the lining of the uterus grows outside of the uterus, often in the pelvic cavity. This can cause inflammation, scarring, and adhesions that lead to significant pain, especially around menstruation. For women trying to conceive, endometriosis can be devastating as it often contributes to infertility.

The endometrial lesions release blood and fluids each month, just like the uterine lining, but the tissue has no way to exit the body. This results in inflammation of surrounding areas like the ovaries, fallopian tubes, and pelvic lining. The buildup of blood and fluids may form cysts known as endometriomas. Scarring and adhesions can distort pelvic anatomy and impact fertility.

Up to 50% of women with endometriosis experience difficulties getting pregnant. The condition can block fallopian tubes, impact egg release, and make conditions inhospitable for implantation or embryo development. Surgery to remove lesions, cysts, and adhesions may improve fertility, but recurrence rates are high. Many women turn to assisted reproductive technologies like IVF to conceive.

The emotional toll of battling endometriosis and infertility can be devastating. Grief over the loss of fertility and dashed hopes each month is compounded by physical suffering. Seeking counseling or joining a support group can help women cope with this painful journey.

Advocating for yourself and finding doctors knowledgeable about endometriosis and infertility is key. While there is no cure, many treatments are available to manage pain, improve quality of life, and enhance fertility. With patience and perseverance, pregnancy is possible, though the road may be long. Staying hopeful in the face of this chronic disease requires tremendous strength and courage.

## The Emotional Toll of Miscarriages and Failed IVF Cycles

The emotional toll of infertility and loss is devastating. Each failed IVF cycle or miscarriage chips away at your hope and optimism.

You pour your heart, soul, energy, and finances into IVF, only to face disappointment again and again. The hormones, procedures and waiting periods are gruelling. With each failure, you can't help but think your dream of becoming a parent is slipping further away.

- The envy and isolation. Seeing pregnancy announcements and baby photos on social media while you struggle in silence. Friends and family don't always understand what you're going through.

- The guilt and self-blame. You start to wonder if there's something wrong with you or if you did something to cause the infertility or losses. This is misplaced guilt - the reality is most cases of infertility and miscarriage are due to biological factors outside of anyone's control.

- The grief. Miscarriages are the loss of a baby, no matter how early, and the grief is real. Failed IVF cycles also represent the loss of hope and a chance at pregnancy. Give yourself space to grieve as needed.

- The strain on relationships. Infertility and loss often impacts couples in different ways and can be a source of tension. Make sure to openly communicate with your partner, set shared expectations, and be each other's support system.

The road to overcoming infertility and loss is a long one, but there are resources and support groups to help you cope during this difficult time. Don't lose hope - stay determined and keep trying. With perseverance, the pain will lessen, and you'll become stronger and wiser, regardless of the outcome. You can get through this.

## Coping With the Grief and Loss of Never Being Able to Have Biological Children

Coping with the grief of never being able to have your own biological children can be an ongoing struggle. As an endometriosis sufferer, you know all too well the physical pain and emotional anguish that comes with battling infertility and pregnancy loss.

### Find Support Groups

Connecting with others who share your experiences can help ease feelings of isolation and provide understanding and comfort. Look for in-person or online support groups for infertility, endometriosis, or infant loss. Speaking with a grief counsellor or therapist who specializes in these areas may also help you work through deep feelings of sadness, anger, or resentment.

**Share Your Story**

Telling your story can be a cathartic release of emotions. Start a blog or vlog to document your journey or look for opportunities to share your experience through support groups, nonprofit organizations, or women's health events. Your story may help other women feel less alone in their struggles and provide hope.

**Practice Self-Care**

Make sure to prioritize your own mental and physical well-being. Exercise, eat healthy, limit alcohol, and get enough sleep. Engage in relaxing activities like yoga, meditation, reading or pursuing a hobby. Take a break from fertility treatments or trying to conceive when you feel overwhelmed. Be kind to yourself and avoid comparing yourself to others.

## Honor Your Loss

For pregnancy loss, consider holding a memorial service, creating a tribute, or starting a ritual to honour your baby's memory on the anniversary of your loss or due date. Naming your baby can help provide closure and acknowledge their brief life. Though the pain may never completely fade, honouring your loss can help the grieving process.

Coping with infertility and infant loss requires patience and compassion. While the pain may always remain, focusing on self-care, finding support, and honouring your experiences can help make the grief more bearable over time. You have endured and will continue to endure. Stay strong in your journey.

## Finding Meaning and Purpose Through Adoption, Fostering, or Childfree Living

After facing infertility and infant loss due to endometriosis, finding meaning and purpose in life again can feel impossible. However, there are options to consider that may help heal your heart.

## Adoption

Adopting a child is a selfless act that provides a loving home for a child in need. Private, foster care, and international adoptions are all possibilities to explore. The adoption process can be long and difficult, but for many women with endometriosis, it is a rewarding path to motherhood.

## Fostering

Fostering children in need provides you an opportunity to nurture, care for and support vulnerable children. While the placement may be temporary, the impact you have on a child's life can be lifelong. Fostering helps address the shortage of available foster parents and provides children stability in a loving home environment.

## Living Childfree

Choosing to live childfree allows you to find purpose and meaning through other avenues. You can devote yourself to your career, creative pursuits, volunteer work, advocacy, or whatever passionate pursuits give you a sense of meaning. While society often pressures women to become mothers, living childfree is a perfectly valid choice. Focusing on self-care, nurturing your relationships, and making a difference in other ways can lead to a life filled with purpose.

The pain of infertility and loss may never completely fade, but in time, the raw ache does become more manageable. Healing looks different for each woman. Seeking counseling or joining a support group can help work through the grieving process. Though the path is difficult, choosing to adopt, foster or live childfree can provide a sense of meaning, purpose, and fulfillment. With each small act of service, each child nurtured, and each life touched, purpose is found again.

**Building a Support System to Help You Through the Dark Days**

Building a support system is crucial when dealing with endometriosis and infertility. Surround yourself with people who understand what you're going through and can provide empathy and comfort.

**Find an endometriosis support group.**

Connecting with others who share your condition can help reduce feelings of isolation. Search online for endometriosis support groups in your area or consider joining an online community. Hearing from others who have been in your shoes and come out the other side can provide much-needed hope.

**Talk to a therapist.**

The emotional toll of battling endometriosis and infertility can be devastating. Speaking with a therapist or counselor who specializes in infertility or chronic illness can help you work through grief, find coping strategies, and maintain your mental health. If in-person therapy isn't an option, look into online services.

**Confide in close friends and family.**

While support groups and therapists are helpful, you also need your close circle of loved ones. Be open with trusted friends and family members about what you're experiencing, both physically and emotionally. Let them know specific ways they can offer support, whether it's just listening without judgment, providing distraction, or helping out with daily tasks.

**Consider joining an infant loss group.**

For those who have experienced miscarriage, stillbirth, or infant death due to endometriosis complications, finding support from others with similar losses can aid in the healing process. Local hospitals, clinics and non-profit organizations often offer support groups and counseling services for bereaved parents. Speaking with others traveling the same heartbreaking path can help reduce feelings of being alone in your grief.

Building this network of support won't make endometriosis or infant loss hurt any less, but surrounding yourself with empathy and compassion can make the dark days a little easier to navigate. Don't isolate yourself during this difficult time — reach out and allow others to support you.

So, you see, the journey of endometriosis is long and painful, both physically and emotionally. But through it all, you persevere. You find strength in community and know that you are not alone in this fight. With each painful period, failed treatment, and longing for a child, you grow stronger and wiser. Endometriosis may have taken away your ability to conceive easily, but it will never take away your resilience and warrior spirit. Though the scars of this illness run deep, you choose each day to stand up and say, "I will not let this disease define me." You are so much more than endometriosis. You are a fighter, a survivor, and a beacon of hope for all those still struggling in the dark. This is your story, your battle, your victory. Endometriosis tried to knock you down, but you found the will to rise up stronger. That is the message of hope to share with others. You are the light that will guide them home.

# 11

## THE ULTIMATE FAIL

This will be the chapter that will upset women the most. I apologize ahead of time. I promise it is an exceedingly difficult and sore subject even for myself. Which is why it needs to be included and addressed. Just hang in there with me, I understand there are women all over the world experiencing the same thing.

As previously mentioned, I had a son back in 2017, two and a half years before I was diagnosed surgically. That pregnancy was by far one of the most difficult things I had ever experienced at the time. Shoot, you think we childhood stressors were stressful. Till you hit adulthood and are fighting tooth and nail to save your baby and do not even understand why your body is so against your pregnancy.

That pregnancy about killed me it seemed. Sounds a bit extreme, I know. Can you imagine how we felt? How my husband may have felt that every time he turned around, I was back in the emergency room being sent to labor and delivery to try to prevent labor? Oh, that was such a stressful time in life. I remember we made it to 36 weeks just barely. He gave birth to a tiny little 5-pound 11 ounce little boy, Parrish. He spent a week in the NICU, as I slowly continued to decline in health. Do you recall earlier I mentioned the problem with weight? Yes, that persists today over 6 years later. I went through highs and lows as far as my health went over the years.

We eventually reached a time where we agreed to try for another baby. As if babies can save marriages, right? About five years went by and we were never successful, our marriage continued to decline. I was miserable and so was he. He never really did understand me or my body. Why I was so sick all the time, or why I was constantly underweight, tired, "lazy", never in the mood. Our marriage struggled for a long time with this. We separated in early 2021 just after New Years.

About 7 months later, I met a man named Alex. Alex has really changed my life in so many ways. He studies Endometriosis and studies my habits and takes the time to try to understand me and how to better help me. This was really the very first time in my life that anyone had taken any real interest or given me a chance to show that I indeed am not a "lazy" soul. I am just exhausted from fighting with something that I really did not even know how to fight. I had just accepted it for what it was.

During the summer of 2022, I had gone to the ER because I was in so much pain. You know the kind if you are a fellow Endo Warrior. You also would know at what level you must be at to force yourself to go to an ER at all. As we all know they are no help whatsoever. Yes, I know you are familiar with that I am referring to. If you do not and you are new to learning what Endometriosis is. Just know we typically have an extremely high pain tolerance. We must darn near be on our death bed type pain before we ever go into any hospital seeking help, because we already know the routine. You get labeled as drug seeking, get told they cannot find anything and that it is in your head, you get made you to believe your crazy and you begin questioning yourself.

This day I had called into work after not being able to sleep for several days and the pain would not let up. Of course, that came with a whole host of problems of its own. As many Endo Warriors know, all too well. Anyway, I went in, and they did all the routine testing and asked if it were possible, I could be pregnant. I said no with full confidence as it has been over 5 years at this point. The test came back positive for pregnancy. I remember feeling a rush of dread come over me. Pure fear. I cried so hard that day. The doctor on shift was so happy but then was confused that I was not sharing the same excitement.

When I say that sense of dread weighed a ton, I mean it was like the entire room was black and I felt so alone and scared. For I already knew what was to come. Well not exactly, but I knew nothing good was to come. I remember calling Alex to inform him of the news. He too was not overly excited. We were really concerned and worried. I think, looking back, that we both in adherently knew on some subconscious level that this would be a short-lived experience and leave us both with apart of our souls broken forever.

I called and resigned my position at the grooming shop, and completely adjusted my life to prepare for that pregnancy. Whatever it would take to ensure he was safe and would make it to term. I tried everything I could. I begged these doctors at every appointment to heed my warning and to pay special attention to this baby. I begged that if something should happen, that I wanted a hysterectomy all together. No matter if he made it or if he did not. It was a part of my afterbirth plans to get that hysterectomy.

I warned and pleaded with every single soul I came across. I do not know why, really. Other than I knew with my first pregnancy my body just was not built for this thing. I knew that Endometriosis was going to make things difficult as it always has. I do not care what the professionals say. They are the ones who say that Endometriosis is "just heavy bleeding and painful cramps". They do not know what they are talking about. They never listen to any women who had endometriosis and blew us off and make us thing we are crazy.

This pregnancy was indeed different. It was easy going and smooth. Aside from constant morning sickness. I grew larger, faster this go around than I did the first time. We even started to get comfortable thinking we were safe. His little heart was always so strong, and he loved to play in the middle of the night when I was trying to sleep. He received his little name, Samuel Adams, after the founding father that is. Alex is a very patriotic, American through and through type individual. Samuel was our little American patriot.

My birthday is October 8th, that weekend was an incredible weekend full of memories and special moments. Alex and the kids (Parrish and his two kids) made me feel so incredibly special. Alex left out on hitch that following Sunday. That following week was awful pain wise; my sciatica was killing me. I did not think much of it, I just did my normal routine to find comfort. I remember making a joke that Sam was hiding in my back as my bump was kind of hiding that day. Again, did not think much of it. That Friday I went to my routine ultrasound, and that day my entire world came crushing down on me.

I wish I were naive and did not know how to read an ultrasound screen, but I do. The tech put the scope on, and I immediately saw it, without her saying a word. She just told me she needed to step out for a moment. My heart sank, I asked my grandma who was there with me that day, "Did you see what I saw?". She replied, "Yes." A whole heap of women came into the room and that further crushed my heart, the nurse looked again and told me I was being admitted because they did not see enough fetal movement.

Again, I already knew. The deep dark secret no one was saying out loud. I already knew. I was scared as my fears were indeed coming true. They made me wait for another two hours before a doctor came in to confirm. I will never forever those piercing words, "Your baby has passed away."

*"Your baby has passed away."*

The entire world fell silent when those words rang out. Even though I already knew and felt prepared for the confirmation. I died in that moment. I gathered myself and started making my phone calls. As it was then time to make decisions. Mine was to go ahead and induce labor and have him that weekend. Alex was in south Texas, thankfully he just so happened to be easy to reach that day. I think I may have already given an incentive that something was not right, so he stayed around to have signal. That has been the most difficult call in my entire life.

My mom and stepdad were there at the hospital within the hour. Seeing the pain on moms' face when she walked in was terrible. As this pregnancy was with a more successful, healthy relationship intact everyone was excited for little Sam. Which was exciting at the time. This day, however, the pain Alex and I shared was spreading to the family in a powerful way. Never has anyone close to any of us experienced what was soon to be labeled as a stillbirth. It never even occurred to us that such a thing could even happen to us.

Mom was standing by the door when she stated that she felt like endometriosis was the cause. As we recall, I mentioned earlier that endometriosis is a little painful lesion that grows around and outside the uterus. The doctor was also standing in the room and stated that "The likelihood of clots being the cause, it just not likely. Endometriosis is typically *excessive bleeding and painful periods.*" To which mom and I shook our head irritated and rolled our eyes. As he walks out, I stated that *this* is always how it goes when you mention anything endometriosis related. They do not listen; they do not care. They are always and have always, thrown out our own subject matter expertise out the window and make us feel like we are losing our minds. Across the board for many if not all endo women.

Mom eventually had to leave and so did my grandma. I sat there by myself for what felt like hours, trying to figure out how I was supposed to do this. I have never made funeral arrangements before. Alex had shared with me that he could not be a part of that, as he was trying to make an 8-hour trip home to be there when Sam was born. I cannot imagine where his mind may have been during that long trip home.

I just knew I needed to prepare and advocate for my son. By this point labor was well on its course. I had picked out the funeral home and made the arrangements for his body. I told them that they were not allowed to perform an autopsy on Sam. However, they could autopsy the placenta. My little brother showed up about 12:00 AM or so and sat with me the entire night. Alex and his mom arrived about 2:00 AM and Sam entered the world at 3:55 AM, October 15th, 2023.

I had just given birth to our beautiful little boy without an epidural and through the most paralyzing fear I had ever experienced. I remember one of my nurses begging me to take her hand as Sam came and the room was dead silent. Whatever was left of that little spark had died by this point. Every ounce of my being was praying, hoping to God that he would magically be born perfectly fine.

To say that I have not struggled with faith since then would be a lie. I understand many women experience this many times over, however, I am not that woman. I struggled with my first pregnancy and this one turned out to not be viable in the end. I already knew my body was not built for this kind of thing, but I tried everything I could because I remained hopeful.

A few days later, the results from the placenta came back. Blood clots all within the umbilical cord and placenta. Yes, you read that right. The very thing that doctor claimed to be so unlikely, turned out to be the very thing that they found. Any medical professional reading this and thinking to yourself, how unlikely this is or that it was caused after his death... I suggest that you take the time to re-educate yourself and do some real research into the matter. The point is to get your attention and encourage someone, anyone, to take endometriosis seriously and do more research and consider our experiences. You will be alarmingly surprised at how many likewise stories you will find.

Meanwhile, everyone collectively agreed to move me to my mom's place while Alex finished up his hitch. Mom has cameras in and out of her house. So, I always had eyes on me. I tend to forget to eat when I am stressed or been through something traumatic. It was a struggle, but I did manage to take care of myself and keep focused on other things. I did, however, spend a lot of time having random breakdowns. It was rough, mentally, truthfully, I was not in a good place. I had myself thinking that I did not deserve to be a mom at all. I struggled with my son Parrish there for a minute afterward.

Alex came home that next Monday, I think. I went home to be with him. I will never forget the kindness he showed me, even though my mind was telling me he hated me, despised me, and blamed me. He showed me love and kindness. We leaned on one another when needed and experienced the range of emotions together. For the first time, I did not feel utterly alone.

The following Wednesday, I was once again admitted into the hospital for emergency surgery. Removal of retained products of birth. Somehow part of the placenta and much of the remaining products left over from birth got left behind. I was so irritatingly annoyed at this point. Embarrassed at the among of blood there was accumulating while they had me in that little gown waiting there, prepping for surgery. I remember when they moved me over to the operating table the horrified looks on these young nurses' faces. I was absolutely mortified. I recall a particular doctor being a part of my surgical team that I had previously plead my case to months prior. He was the very first doctor to see me for a prenatal visit. I cannot describe the amount of hatred and loathing I left for this man. Not to mention going like a week and a half, profusely bleeding out from left over placenta and pregnancy products.

I came home to a house full of kids that evening. Alex's kids and my oldest boy were home that day. From the mental aspect of things, this was exceedingly difficult to be around. I just wanted to be alone, I was sore from both birth and surgery still. I was beyond exhausted. Mastitis was beginning to kick in triple time. The kids of course had no inkling of what had happened the week before. Other than "baby brother died in mommy's tummy", that was like a spear to the heart, hearing that. Those days dragged on and on. The emotional roller coaster was chaotic and lonely. Fortunately, Alex was so tuned that he knew if I disappeared it was because I was hiding somewhere crying my eyes out. He would come to find me and tell me to lean into him, that we were both feeling the pain and that it was important to lean into one another, reminding me that I in fact am not alone.

---

Fetuses and neonates of women with endometriosis were also more likely to have preterm premature rupture of membranes, preterm birth, small for gestational age < 10th percentile, NICU admission, stillbirths, and neonatal death. Maternal endometriosis had borderline association with infant low birth weight <2500 g (Lalani et al., 2018).[6]

---

[6] Lalani, S., Choudhry, A. J., Firth, B., Bacal, Walker, M., Wen, S. P., Singh, S. K., Amath, A., Hodge, M., & Chen, I. (2018). Endometriosis and adverse maternal, fetal and neonatal outcomes, a systematic review and meta-analysis. Human Reproduction, 33(10), 1854–1865. https://doi.org/10.1093/humrep/dey269

# 12

PERSONAL LESSONS

I think as women, when we experience a loss of this magnitude, we forget that we have spouses going through the same experiences. However, as men, they handle themselves in a fashion that makes them look invincible thus making us feel alone and not really realizing that they too are feeling the pain and loss. It comes out in diverse ways for them. They will sit there and tell you to cry onto them while they hold you, while they are the ones going off by themselves to release that emotion. What I learned during this experience is that everyone, my brother who was there that night, the grandparents on both sides and anyone actively involved were all incredibly deeply affected. While in the moment we as women are going through a series of emotions that make you feel like your soul is being ripped out of your body. Your brain telling you all the deep dark nasty comments and thoughts, convincing you that you are to blame and that everyone hates you; that you are undeserving.

What I have also learned during this time is that women who experience miscarriage or infertility of any form, often go through the similar emotions. Self-doubt, self-loathing, tearing ourselves down from the inside out. Not every story is similar, each individual story is different and unique, many women experience these things in complete loneliness. Some even repeat the process over and over in hopes of finally landing that healthy, beautiful baby. This book is really angled at endometriosis, but while we are on the topic we will explore women's health, and several topics like this one in its entirety. As to not take away from any others going through something similar. I am not saying endometriosis is the only cause of infertility or loss, it is just an additional factor that society fails to acknowledge.

Just as society fails to acknowledge that postpartum depression is real. Not all women experience such a thing. To those who have never seen it for themselves, they believe it is as real as a unicorn. The fact of the matter is that it is very real, and it takes lives every day. Endometriosis along with the mental teardown it brings with it, has taken lives. Lack thereof in women rights among other things.

I read every single day in Endometriosis, PCOS and Adenomyosis groups on social media that women worldwide are experiencing infertility and loss. It is astounding how many likewise stories come out talking about the lack thereof in rights and compassion from medical professionals. It is furthermore alarming the number of women worldwide currently living in a state of mind of no hope, despair and on the verge of wanting to just give up at life. You can feel the anger and sadness coming through the forum.

It is comforting in a way to realize you are not alone in your fight with any of these diseases. Especially for me, endometriosis. It is so widely unknown and unfamiliar that many doctors have no idea what it even is in the U.S. anyway. Thus, is where the generic definition keeps coming up. As I do more research for this book, I find more research done outside of the U.S. proving all my points to be fact. Afterall, I do live inside of this body and have been fighting this fight for almost 20 years now.

To recap, endometriosis is when the menstrual blood flows backwards up and out the fallopian tubes into the body cavity (retrograde menstruation). The blood has nowhere to go, the body absorbs it and lesions form on the outside of the uterus, along organs, and sometimes imbed into muscle tissue. When they burst or are removed, scar tissue then grows in its place. These lesions can grow back on the scar tissue. Lesions can spread and cause havoc all over the body. Every cycle the lesions bleed just the same as you would on your cycle. The body absorbs it, and the cycle continues. We experience what is known as an Endo Flair up. During a flair up many women experience extreme abdominal swelling, lower back, and hip pain.

Depending on the severity some may feel pain down their legs so debilitating that it is extremely difficult to move. Migraines, nausea, and vomiting. Excessive, heavy bleeding, very painful labor like cramps that put labor itself to shame on the pain scale. The list goes on and on. If you went to Dr. Google, then you would find some generic condensed version that leaves out a lot of what is mentioned here.

Endometriosis, among other known diseases, causes infertility by growing on the ovaries or fallopian tubes and destroying them. Even in my case with the cysts that grow on my ovaries. As I observe and do my own research, I find more and more women learning they are infertile do to some sort of abruption to their reproductive organs. Many did go to the ER initially with pain that the medical professionals could not diagnose and were sent home with no help. Just to later find out that they had a fallopian tube or ovary abrupt. I have seen cases where the scar tissue caused blockages, others were hormone related.

Research further shows that endometrial cells can spread by contaminating other healthy cells elsewhere in the body (transformation of peritoneal cells), as the Mayo Clinic[7] states. They are even saying that there is a possibility of embryonic cell transformation, where hormones such as estrogen may transform embryonic cells into endometrial-like cell implants during puberty (Endometriosis - Symptoms and Causes - Mayo Clinic, 2018).

My favorite, that I was told was happening to me personally, was that the endometrial cells were implanting into old scar tissue and into old surgical scars. Mayo Clinic also goes on to say that endometriosis is classified as an immune system disorder. I 100% believe endometriosis attacks the entire immune system. The fact that the disease attacks all reproductive organs, the bowel, the abdominal cavity along with other organs and surrounding muscle tissue, and even has been found in the lungs and brain strongly suggests so. The effects it has on our mental state, migraines, and pain all over the entire body; enough to be debilitating and make us physically sick. Strongly

---

[7] Endometriosis - Symptoms and causes - Mayo Clinic. (2018, July 24). Mayo Clinic. https://www.mayoclinic.org/diseases-conditions/endometriosis/symptoms-causes/syc-20354656

suggest that the disease is far more than just bad cramps and heavy bleeding as the doctors like to say.

The surreal impact this disease has on all our lives is unbelievable. It is quite astonishing the fact that our trusted medical providers refuse to listen to our pleas, letting us suffer for years and years. It is disheartening to read day after day the pleas of women all over the world experiencing the same hopelessness and pain as I am.

What is even more interesting is that there is such a thing as 'Silent Endometriosis'. In the event of silent endometriosis, the patient gets accidentally diagnosed and usually is covered in the disease and never even knew it. They never feel pain, they never had any abnormal cycles, I believe the most they have experienced was a form of infertility which led to exploratory surgery to begin with. Sometimes it has even been discovered during other non-related surgeries.

It really is no wonder why this disease is so baffling to so many. Nonetheless, this is no reason or excuse as to why we should not be heard or listened to. Let us talk about women's rights, we will go into further detail in a later chapter but get this; when I found out I was pregnant with my second son, it was just days before the Roe v. Wade law was overturned. Never did that law ever matter to me before, it never occurred to me as it would directly affect me. I was under the impression it ONLY mattered to those who 'wanted' abortions.

I soon learned that it had everything to do with us as women. I found myself in the unique situation where had if I made the decision to terminate due to medical reasons, I'd have to travel several states over. I will explain later why this has become a direct problem for me.

From a medical standpoint, it all started to make sense as to why that law was so important to women's rights. I do not think it was originally put in place for those women out there who disrespect the system. Even though that is what the media wants you to think. I realized having laws in place to protect our rights if a medical emergency occurs with pregnancy, women are not forced to carry their deceased or unviable baby to term.

# PART 3

FDA AND MEDICAL PROFESSIONALS

# 13

# ENDOMETRIOSIS DESERVES MORE FROM THE FDA

The FDA has only approved a handful of treatments, most with serious side effects, and no cure. It's time for the FDA to make endometriosis a higher priority and support research into new treatment options for this debilitating disease. Women's pain is not "normal" or "in their heads." Endometriosis deserves more from the FDA.

[8]The FDA currently recognizes endometriosis as a benign gynecological condition, despite the severe impacts it has on quality of life for those affected. As a result, treatments are regulated as medical devices or drugs, limiting innovation.[9]

The FDA approves endometriosis treatments like hormonal contraceptives, pain medications, and surgeries based primarily on their safety and efficacy in managing symptoms. However, they do little to address the underlying condition. Promising new treatments take years of testing to reach the market, even as endometriosis continues progressing in patients.

Advocacy groups are lobbying the FDA to reclassify endometriosis as a chronic disease to spur development of disease-modifying treatments. This could incentivize research into the mechanisms driving endometriosis progression and allow faster approval of

---

[8] "Myovant Sciences and Pfizer Receive U.S. FDA Approval ...": https://www.pfizer.com/news/press-release/press-release-detail/myovant-sciences-and-pfizer-receive-us-fda-approval

[9] "A Clinician's Guide to the Treatment of Endometriosis with ...": https://www.ncbi.nlm.nih.gov/pmc/articles/PMC8064963/

treatments targeting the condition itself, not just symptoms.

Patients also argue that quality of life measures should play a larger role in the FDA's evaluations, given the life-altering impacts of endometriosis like pain, infertility, and lost work or school days. Broader measures of treatment efficacy may encourage development of therapies providing meaningful relief and control of the disease in the long run.

While reclassification and changes to the approval process will take time, continued advocacy is critical to driving the systemic changes needed to improve treatment options and quality of life for the millions of women living with endometriosis. The FDA has an opportunity to become a true partner in the fight against this chronic and debilitating disease.

The FDA plays a crucial role in medical research and approval of new treatments, yet endometriosis receives disproportionately little attention. Endometriosis affects over 6.5 million women in the U.S., yet the FDA has only approved a few treatments, and none are highly effective. [10]

Endometriosis causes debilitating pain, infertility, and other life-altering symptoms, but its exact causes and progression remain poorly understood. The FDA should prioritize research into the origins and mechanisms of this complex disease. Additional studies could uncover new treatment targets and lead to non-invasive diagnostics.

The average woman sees five doctors over seven years before receiving an endometriosis diagnosis. The FDA should evaluate new screening tools to reduce diagnosis time and prevent years of needless suffering. Earlier detection and treatment can slow disease progression and reduce long-term complications.

Existing endometriosis treatments often cause intolerable side effects and fail to provide long-term relief. The FDA's guidelines for approving new drugs are too rigid for a disease as variable as endometriosis. Flexible, patient-centered approval processes are

---

[10] "Pharmaceuticals targeting signaling pathways of ...": https://www.ncbi.nlm.nih.gov/pmc/articles/PMC8252000/

needed to make new treatments available, especially for severe, hard-to-treat cases.

Women deserve more options than repeated surgeries or drugs with limited benefit and harsh side effects. The FDA has the power to change and save lives through promoting innovative endometriosis research and groundbreaking new treatments. It's time endometriosis gets the attention and action it demands. Millions of women are counting on progress.

The FDA regulates drugs and medical devices in the U.S., including those used to diagnose and treat endometriosis. Increased involvement and oversight from the FDA could help improve care for endometriosis in several ways:

**Accelerating Approval of New Treatments**

The FDA evaluates new drugs and devices to ensure they are safe and effective before approving them for use. Expediting the approval process for promising endometriosis treatments could help make them available to patients sooner. The FDA offers programs like Fast Track, Breakthrough Therapy, and Accelerated Approval to speed up approval for drugs that meet certain criteria. Applying these programs to endometriosis treatments may allow new options to reach the market faster.

## Encouraging Research and Development

The FDA not only approves new treatments but also provides guidance to companies during the research and development process. By making endometriosis a priority, the FDA could offer incentives for companies to invest in researching new diagnostics, drugs, and medical devices for endometriosis. This may motivate more companies to pursue endometriosis as an area of focus, ultimately resulting in more treatment options for patients.

## Improving Patient Education

The FDA reviews and approves patient education materials to ensure information is accurate, balanced, and helpful. Requiring companies to provide comprehensive patient education about endometriosis treatments could help address common issues like unrealistic expectations, lack of disease understanding, and knowledge gaps about risks and benefits. This may enable patients to have more informed discussions with their doctors about the best options for their situation.

In summary, the FDA wields significant influence over the development and availability of medical treatments. Applying this influence to endometriosis could spur progress that dramatically improves the landscape of care and support for endometriosis patients in the coming years. By making endometriosis a priority, providing incentives and guidance to companies, and improving patient education, the FDA may be able to positively impact endometriosis at a regulatory level.

You now understand the lack of progress in endometriosis treatment options despite the FDA's role in regulating them. The time is now to demand more funding, support, and urgency around this debilitating condition that affects millions of women. Contact your political representatives and the FDA to express your concerns. Join advocacy groups raising awareness of endometriosis and put pressure on institutions with the power to accelerate diagnosis, treatment, and eventually a cure. While the road ahead remains long, together we can give endometriosis the attention and resources it deserves so that someday women will have more options and hope. The power is in your hands—use your voice to inspire change.

# 14

## ENDOMETRIOSOS TREATMENT DEVELOPMENT: THE CHALLENGES OF FDA REGULATION

Unfortunately, the road to new endometriosis therapies is long and difficult. The FDA requires extensive testing to ensure new drugs are safe and effective before approving them for public use. While crucial for patient well-being, this process significantly slows the pace at which promising new endometriosis treatments to become available. Researchers face many hurdles proving a treatment works and deserves FDA approval. Though the future looks promising, the wait continues.

Developing new treatments requires extensive research and clinical trials to ensure safety and efficacy before approval by the FDA. This process typically takes 10-15 years and over $1 billion. For endometriosis, the challenges are many:

Lack of non-invasive diagnostic tools make early diagnosis and treatment difficult. New imaging techniques and biomarkers are needed.

The cause of endometriosis remains unknown, complicating the search for new treatment targets. Research into the role of genetics, hormones, immune system dysfunction, and environmental factors is ongoing.

Obtaining research funding and interest from pharmaceutical companies has been an uphill battle given the "orphan disease" status. Grassroots efforts by advocacy groups have helped raise awareness.

Clinical trial recruitment is challenging due to invasive surgeries often required for diagnosis, as well as a lack of standardized evaluation methods to determine treatment efficacy. Patient reported outcome measures may help.

FDA approval requires demonstrating a statistically significant impact on symptoms like pain, fertility, and quality of life. This can be difficult given the variability in women's experiences with endometriosis.

Continued research and advocacy are critical to overcoming these barriers. By understanding the challenges in developing and approving new treatments, we can support efforts to find better options for managing this enigmatic disease. The women suffering from endometriosis deserve nothing less.

Getting a new treatment approved by the FDA is a long and complex process. As a patient, it can feel frustrating waiting for new options, but regulation helps ensure safety and efficacy.

For new drugs, companies must first conduct preclinical testing on animals to determine if it's reasonably safe for humans. If results are promising, companies submit an Investigational New Drug application to start clinical trials in humans.

**Clinical trials occur in three phases:**

Phase I tests the drug on a small group of people to evaluate safety and dosage.

Phase II expands testing to several hundred people to assess effectiveness and side effects.

Phase III trials can include thousands of people across multiple sites to confirm effectiveness, monitor side effects, and compare to existing treatments.

If trials are successful, companies submit a New Drug Application detailing all testing and results. The FDA reviews applications to determine if the benefits outweigh the risks. Only then may the drug be approved for marketing.

Endometriosis treatments face additional hurdles. The condition is complex with symptoms varying between individuals. Large scale trials are difficult and expensive. Many investigational drugs have been abandoned mid-trial or rejected by the FDA.

While the approval process takes time, it helps guarantee new treatments are safe and effective for this debilitating disease. With continued research and advocacy, more options will emerge to provide relief for all sufferers.

Endometriosis clinical trials face many challenges due to FDA regulations. The FDA requires strict protocols for approving new treatments to ensure safety and efficacy. However, these regulations can slow the process.

Recruiting women with endometriosis to participate in clinical trials is difficult. Endometriosis impacts an estimated 1 in 10 women, but many remain undiagnosed for years. Those who are diagnosed may be reluctant to participate due to the demanding nature of trials, discomfort with experimenting on their bodies, or distrust in the medical system.

The FDA often requires placebo control groups in trials to determine a treatment's effectiveness. However, denying women an actual treatment for a painful condition raises ethical concerns. The placebo effect also tends to be high in endometriosis trials due to the subjective nature of pain, making results harder to interpret.

The FDA emphasizes objective measures and standardized outcomes, like reduced lesion size. But endometriosis pain and quality of life are highly individualized and complex. What works for one woman may not help another. Focusing on narrow outcomes risks missing meaningful benefits.

Conducting clinical trials is an expensive, years-long process. The high costs and uncertainty of FDA approval discourage some pharmaceutical companies from investing in endometriosis research. For those that do, the long timeline means new treatments can take over a decade to reach women who need them.

While rigorous testing of new treatments is crucial, the challenges of FDA regulation in endometriosis highlight the need for alternative trial designs, outcome measures tailored to patient experiences, and policies incentivizing continued progress in this underserved area of women's health. With creativity and compassion, researchers and regulators can work together to accelerate safe and effective new options for the millions of women living with this disease.

When developing new treatments for endometriosis, pharmaceutical companies and researchers face many challenges in gaining approval from the U.S. Food and Drug Administration (FDA). The FDA regulates drugs and medical devices in the U.S. to ensure safety and effectiveness before they reach the market. For endometriosis, the complex nature of the condition and limited treatment options create unique difficulties in the regulatory process.

Endometriosis manifests in many different ways for each patient. The FDA requires clinical trials to prove a treatment's efficacy, but finding a large enough sample size of women with similar symptoms is difficult. Treatments also may impact women differently depending on factors like age, ethnicity, and the locations of endometrial-like tissue. Designing trials that account for this variability and heterogeneity poses problems.

There are currently few approved treatment options for endometriosis, so new therapies aim to fill an unmet need. However, the FDA often has higher safety standards for first-in-class drugs or treatments without comparable medications already on the market. While the intention is to protect patients, these standards can make gaining approval more challenging and prolong the process. For endometriosis, the potential benefits of new treatment options must be balanced with safety to determine if the risks outweigh the rewards.

Even after clinical trials demonstrate safety and efficacy, the regulatory process for endometriosis therapies typically takes many years. On average, new drugs that make it to market can take over a decade of research and development. For endometriosis, treatments may take even longer to account for the complex nature of the disease and lack of approved comparators. While a long approval process aims to protect patients, it also means much-needed new treatment options are delayed in reaching women who could benefit from them.

In summary, endometriosis poses unique challenges in the development and approval of new treatments due to its heterogeneity, limited treatment options currently available, and a prolonged regulatory process. Still, continued research and advocacy offer hope for improved care and management of this painful condition in the future.

To accelerate approval of new endometriosis treatments, collaboration between advocacy groups, researchers, and the FDA is key. Working together, they can design trials that generate meaningful data and navigate the regulatory process more efficiently.

Advocacy organizations like the Endometriosis Foundation of America (EFA) and the Endometriosis Association (EA) support people with endometriosis and fund research. They understand patients' unmet needs and priorities for new treatments. The EFA's Scientific Advisory Board and EA's Medical Advisory Board include leading doctors and researchers. These groups can provide input on trial designs to ensure new treatments target what really matters to patients. They can also help recruit trial participants from their community.

Researchers at universities, hospitals and biopharmaceutical companies develop new treatment approaches and conduct clinical trials. Close collaboration with advocacy groups and regulators helps ensure their work will translate into approved options for patients. The FDA provides guidance on trial designs and endpoints to meet their standards of safety and efficacy. Researchers may get faster approval by focusing trials on patient-centric outcomes and quality-of-life measures that advocacy groups recommend.

The FDA aims to approve new drugs and devices efficiently while upholding high standards for safety and effectiveness. Although the approval process can seem slow, the FDA is working to speed the development and review of treatments for conditions like endometriosis that lack good options. They provide various resources to help sponsors design trials that will generate data for approval decisions. Meeting with researchers and patient groups helps the FDA understand what new treatments and trial outcomes will benefit those with endometriosis.

Through collaborative efforts, advocacy groups, researchers and regulators can find common ground and solutions to address the challenges of developing and approving innovative endometriosis treatments. Patients deserve more and better options, and by working together, the path forward can be expedited.

So, while the road to new endometriosis treatments is long, progress is being made. The key is advocating for continued research funding and pushing the FDA to consider the lived experiences of women with this condition. Though regulation is necessary, over-regulation risks cutting off the pipeline of new options before they have a chance to reach those who need them most. Staying informed and engaged as new clinical trials emerge is one of the most impactful actions any woman can take. Though endometriosis may not yet have a cure, every new treatment brings us one step closer to a future where fewer women suffer in silence. There is still hope - we just have to keep fighting for it.

# 15

## THE LONG ROAD TO DIAGNOSIS: HOW THE MEDICAL SYSTEM FAILS ENDOMETRIOSIS PAITENTS

Doctors frequently minimize or ignore symptoms, leaving many to suffer through a prolonged diagnostic journey. This failure highlights deep flaws in how the medical system treats women and understands conditions like endometriosis that primarily impact female reproductive health. Your pain is real, and you deserve answers. It's time we demand better understanding, treatment, and support for this all-too-common disease. The long road to a diagnosis has taken enough casualties already.

## The Difficulty of Diagnosing Endometriosis

The average time for an endometriosis diagnosis is 7-10 years. Why does it take so long? There are a few reasons the medical system fails endometriosis patients:

- **Lack of Knowledge**

Many doctors simply don't know enough about endometriosis or don't consider it as a possible diagnosis. They often attribute symptoms like painful periods, chronic pelvic pain, and painful intercourse to "normal" menstrual issues or gastrointestinal problems.

- Endometriosis education is limited in medical schools, so new doctors start their careers with little knowledge about this complex disease.

- Doctors rely on outdated ideas about endometriosis, like the myth that it only affects women in their 30s-40s or that pain is linked to the menstrual cycle.

- **Dismissal of Women's Pain**

   Women's pain and symptoms are often normalized, dismissed, or misdiagnosed. Doctors frequently tell endometriosis patients that severe pain with their period is "normal" or that they're being "dramatic." This systemic dismissal and lack of trust in women's self-reports delays diagnosis and treatment.

- **Inadequate Diagnostic Tools**

   The only way to definitively diagnose endometriosis is through laparoscopic surgery. This requires general anesthesia and a surgical procedure to visualize the pelvis. Many doctors are hesitant to refer patients for surgery without "concrete" evidence from less-invasive tests, even though these tests often miss endometriosis. This results in patients suffering for years before getting the surgery that finally leads to a diagnosis and treatment.

The road to an endometriosis diagnosis is long and difficult. But with increased awareness, improved medical education, and more willingness to trust and act on women's pain reports, patients may get the answers and treatment they need much sooner.

- **Doctor Dismissiveness and Delayed Diagnosis**

When you first start experiencing painful periods, nausea, fatigue, and other symptoms, you hope your doctor will take your concerns seriously and help determine the cause. Unfortunately, for endometriosis patients, the road to diagnosis is often long and frustrating.[11]

Doctors frequently dismiss or downplay women's menstrual health issues. They may blame symptoms on factors like stress or hormones rather than investigating

---

[11] https://endometriosisnews.com/2019/04/12/patients-give-up-work-system-fails/

https://bmcwomenshealth.biomedcentral.com/articles/10.1186/s12905-022-01603-6

further. Some physicians still cling to the outdated notion that extreme menstrual pain is "normal". As a result, the average endometriosis diagnosis takes up to 10 years

During this prolonged quest for answers, patients are typically offered temporary solutions like birth control pills, NSAIDs or surgery for ovarian cysts. While these may provide some relief, they do not treat the underlying endometriosis. Patients continue suffering through a diminished quality of life with limited treatment options and little hope.

When a diagnosis is finally made, damage has already been done with endometrial lesions possibly infiltrating other organs. Yet some physicians remain reluctant to consider endometriosis a chronic disease requiring long-term management. They may recommend another temporary solution instead of excision surgery and hormonal therapy known to effectively ease symptoms.

Endometriosis patients deserve doctors who listen, provide compassionate care and stay up-to-date with the latest treatment approaches. When the medical system fails us, we must be our own best advocates in seeking out knowledgeable specialists and demanding the care we need. Our health and lives depend on it.

- **The Physical and Emotional Toll of Undiagnosed Endometriosis**

The physical and emotional effects of undiagnosed endometriosis can be devastating. You've lived with excruciating pain and discomfort for years without answers or relief. The uncertainty, doubt, and disregard from doctors have taken their toll.

- **Unrelenting Pain**

The chronic pelvic pain, cramping, and stabbing sensations make it hard to function. Pain that leaves you unable to work, go to school, or socialize is not normal. Heavy, prolonged periods worsen the agony. You dread that "time of the month" and what fresh hell each cycle may bring.

- **Hopelessness and Isolation**

Being told repeatedly that the pain is "in your head" or "just part of being a woman" breeds feelings of hopelessness, self-doubt, and isolation. Friends and family don't understand why you cancel plans or can't keep up. You start to wonder if the doctors are right and you're just being dramatic or hysterical. This cycle of suffering and dismissal leaves deep emotional wounds.

- **Anxiety and Depression**

Living with an undiagnosed chronic illness for years inflicts psychological distress. You develop anxiety over when the next flare-up may strike and how bad it will be. The lack of validation, answers or treatment may plunge you into depression. Your mental health and relationships suffer, compounding the physical issues.

Getting the correct endometriosis diagnosis is essential to breaking this cycle, accessing proper treatment, and reclaiming your life. Though the road is long, find doctors who listen, connect with support groups, and don't lose hope. You deserve to feel heard, understood, and helped. Staying determined in your search for answers will lead to the care and relief you need. There are more and better solutions available than you've been led to believe. You are not alone in this fight.

- **Seeking Alternative Opinions and Self-Advocacy**

When doctors dismiss your symptoms or tell you the pain is normal, it can be frustrating and make you feel unheard. Many endometriosis patients face obstacles in getting an accurate diagnosis and finding the right treatment. Don't lose hope—there are steps you can take to advocate for yourself and get the care you deserve.

- **Seek Second Opinions**

If your doctor brushes off your concerns or says there's nothing wrong, get another perspective. Do some research to find an endometriosis specialist in your area and schedule a consultation. Come prepared to discuss your full medical history and specific symptoms. A specialist may be more likely to recognize the signs of endometriosis and suggest appropriate testing.

- **Do Your Own Research**

Unfortunately, some doctors receive little training about endometriosis and may not fully understand the condition. Educate yourself on the latest treatments, diagnostic tools, and management options so you can have an informed discussion with your doctor. Check reputable sources like the Endometriosis Foundation of America, Endometriosis.org, and peer-reviewed studies. The more you know about the disease, the better equipped you'll be to advocate for the care you need.

- **Push for Diagnostic Testing**

If pain medication and birth control are not relieving your symptoms, ask your doctor about diagnostic tests like pelvic exams, ultrasounds, or laparoscopies to determine if endometriosis or other conditions are present. Be your own best advocate by speaking up about how the pain impacts your life and that you want to get to the root cause of the problem. Don't stop seeking answers until you have a definitive diagnosis and treatment plan.

- **Find the Right Doctor for You**

Getting the right doctor on your side, one who listens and wants to help relieve your suffering, can make all the difference in properly diagnosing and managing endometriosis. You may need to see several physicians before finding someone you fully trust and connect with. Once you do, you'll have an ally to partner with on the long road to wellness. Stay strong in your journey—there are caring doctors out there and hope for a better future.

## Creating Change: How the Medical Community Can Better Support Patients

The medical community has a long way to go to properly diagnose and treat endometriosis. Too often, patients are dismissed, misdiagnosed, and left without adequate care or support. Things need to change.

- **Listen and Believe Patients**

The first step is for doctors to listen to and believe patients about their symptoms. Endometriosis can take over a decade to diagnose because symptoms are often dismissed as "normal" menstrual pain or discomfort. Doctors must trust that patients know their own bodies and pain levels.

- **Improve Diagnostic Process**

The current diagnosing process relies on invasive surgeries like laparoscopies to visually confirm the presence of endometriosis. This needs improvement. Developing a simple blood test to detect endometriosis bio-markers could help reduce diagnosis time. Doctors also need better training to spot signs of endometriosis in initial exams and refer patients to specialists sooner.

- **Expand Treatment Options**

Treatment options are limited for endometriosis. Hormone therapies and surgeries are commonly prescribed but often fail to provide long-term relief or do not work for all patients. The medical community must invest in developing alternative treatments like improved hormonal contraceptives as well as evaluating natural remedies. They should also make emerging options like magnetic resonance guided focused ultrasound readily available and covered by insurance.

- **Provide Ongoing Support**

Endometriosis is a chronic illness, so doctors must offer ongoing support for patients. This includes managing side effects of treatments, monitoring progression, and helping patients cope with symptoms that persist or return. Doctors should connect patients with endometriosis support groups and make mental health resources readily available. Patients need to be heard, supported, and cared for.

The medical system fails endometriosis patients in so many ways, but through listening, believing, improving diagnosis and treatment, and providing ongoing support, real change can happen. Patients deserve nothing less. Together, doctors and patients can work to find solutions so endometriosis is no longer the "invisible illness."

After all the years of pain and suffering, you finally have answers. But the relief is bittersweet. Why did it take so long? Why were your pleas for help ignored for over a decade? The medical system failed you, and it fails countless others with endometriosis each and every day. But now you have a diagnosis, a community for support, and treatment options to explore.

The road was long and difficult, but you persevered. You advocated for yourself when no one else would. And though the scars of dismissals and misdiagnoses still linger, you now look to the future with the knowledge and voice to help make change.

Endometriosis may be a lifelong condition, but no longer will you suffer in silence. Your story and your advocacy can help ensure others get the care and answers they deserve. The road ahead remains long, but at last there is hope.

# PART 4

## DALLAS BUYERS CLUB

**\*\*IF YOU HAVEN'T ALREADY YOU SHOULD WATCH THE DALLAS BUYERS CLUB TO UNDERSTAND THE COORILATION BEING MADE HERE\*\***

# 16

## HIV/AIDS AND ENDOMETRIOSIS: DECADES APART BUT STILL FIGHTING THE SAME FIGHT

There are few medical conditions that have faced more challenges than HIV/AIDS and endometriosis. HIV/AIDS emerged in the 1980s as a frightening and misunderstood disease that was stigmatized and politicized. Today, endometriosis affects over 176 million women worldwide, yet it remains underfunded, misdiagnosed, and poorly understood. Despite being separated by decades, those living with HIV/AIDS in the 1980s and women currently living with endometriosis are united by parallel struggles. Both have had to fight for visibility, push back against stigma, and demand better treatment options and a cure. This chapter examines the similarities in the experiences faced by these two communities in their fights for recognition, funding, and improved health outcomes. Though the medical conditions differ, the battles against marginalization and neglect remain the same.

- **The Early Days of the HIV/AIDS Epidemic in the 1980s**

When HIV/AIDS first emerged in the early 1980s, medical professionals were unsure of how it was transmitted or how to properly contain it. The early days of the epidemic were filled with fear, stigma, and misinformation.

- **Lack of Understanding**

Initially, the scientific and medical communities did not fully understand HIV/AIDS. They knew it impacted the immune system but were unsure of how it was transmitted from person to person. This lack of understanding led to the belief that it could be spread through casual contact. As a result, those with HIV/AIDS faced discrimination and ostracization.

- **Stigma and Misinformation**

The unknowns surrounding transmission led to rampant stigma against groups like homosexual men, who were disproportionately impacted early on. People feared contracting HIV/AIDS from casual contact with those infected. This stigma was compounded by moral judgements against groups associated with the virus. Public misconceptions were widespread before public health campaigns educated people on how HIV/AIDS is actually transmitted through direct blood contact, sexual activity, and needle sharing.

- **Fighting for Recognition and Resources**

Advocacy groups had to fight for funding, research, and recognition of the epidemic. They lobbied governments for resources and support, organized protests, and campaigns to raise awareness, and spread accurate information about the virus. Groups like ACT UP were on the frontlines pushing for access to promising new medications and a faster government response. Through their tireless efforts, views gradually shifted, and life-saving treatments were developed. But for those suffering in the early days, the fight was long and arduous.

Decades later, though much progress has been made, the experience of women with endometriosis today in some ways mirrors the early struggles of the HIV/AIDS community. There are still misunderstandings, lack of knowledge in the medical field, and difficulties getting a proper diagnosis and treatment. However, by learning from the past, perhaps the endometriosis community can find strength and inspiration to persevere against similar obstacles. Together, step by step, through advocacy and action, changes can be achieved.

- **Stigma and Misinformation Surrounding HIV/AIDS**

In the early days of the HIV/AIDS epidemic, a lack of scientific understanding about the disease led to widespread stigma and misinformation. Many saw HIV/AIDS as a "gay disease" or divine punishment, creating discrimination against the LGBTQ community. This stigma prevented open discussion and slowed research efforts.

Public health initiatives were met with resistance due to moral objections and fear of the unknown. Educational campaigns had limited success, as misconceptions about transmission and treatment abounded. The medical community itself was divided, with some doctors refusing to treat HIV/AIDS patients.

Women with endometriosis face similar challenges today. Endometriosis remains poorly understood, leading to myths that it is rare or "just bad cramps." Due to societal taboos around menstruation and women's health issues, endometriosis is often not discussed openly. This contributes to the average 7-10 years delay in diagnosis, allowing the condition to worsen untreated.

Doctors frequently dismiss or misdiagnose endometriosis, demonstrating a lack of knowledge and empathy regarding a disease that impacts over 11% of women. Women report feeling stigmatized or that they are not believed due to stereotypical views of gender and pain. Under-researched and under-funded, endometriosis receives a fraction of the research funding of similarly prevalent diseases.

Decades apart, HIV/AIDS and endometriosis sufferers have fought against stigma, misinformation, and discrimination to gain recognition, research, and treatment for their life-altering conditions. Through the courageous efforts of activists and advocates, progress has been won, but the fight is not over. Understanding and open discussion of these diseases remains key to improving outcomes and quality of life for all.

- **Difficulty Accessing Healthcare for People With HIV/AIDS**

In the early days of the HIV/AIDS epidemic, those diagnosed faced enormous challenges in accessing healthcare. Discrimination and stigmatization were widespread, with many in the medical community refusing to treat HIV/AIDS patients. Lack of knowledge about the disease and how it spread also led to misconceptions that fueled fear and prejudice.

People living with HIV/AIDS had trouble finding physicians and clinics willing to provide them care. When they did gain access, the prohibitively high cost of early antiretroviral drugs and treatments placed them out of reach for most. Government inaction and inadequate funding for research further exacerbated these barriers. Many of those afflicted could not afford private insurance and did not qualify for government assistance.

Today, similar difficulties in accessing medical care persist for women with endometriosis. While not contagious, endometriosis is also a complex disease that is poorly understood, leading to delays in diagnosis and mismanagement of symptoms. Patients frequently report encountering physicians who dismiss or minimize their complaints, attributing them to normal menstruation.

The average woman sees five doctors over eight years before receiving an endometriosis diagnosis, while an estimated 40-60% remain undiagnosed. Treatment options are limited, and excision surgery with an expert endometriosis surgeon is considered the gold standard yet is not widely available or covered by most insurance plans. The annual cost of endometriosis care in the U.S. is approximately $50 billion, leaving many unable to get the treatment they need.

Decades apart, those with HIV/AIDS and endometriosis have faced parallel struggles in overcoming stigma, lack of research, and barriers to affordable, specialized care. While progress has been made, ongoing advocacy is still required to ensure equitable access to healthcare for these vulnerable populations. Both diseases highlight the need to reduce the stigma surrounding chronic illnesses and women's health issues.

- **The Fight for Recognition and Research Funding for HIV/AIDS**

In the early 1980s, HIV/AIDS emerged as a new disease that caused a weakened immune system and rare cancers in young, otherwise healthy individuals. However, due to the populations initially impacted, including gay men and intravenous drug users, HIV/AIDS was stigmatized and largely ignored.

Advocacy groups had to fight to raise awareness of this new disease and gain recognition from health organizations, political leaders, and society. It took years of activism and lobbying for HIV/AIDS to be declared a national health crisis in the U.S. Additionally, these groups had to push for increased research funding to better understand HIV, how it spread, and develop treatments. Federal research funding for HIV/AIDS grew slowly in the 1980s, despite the increasing death toll.

Today, women with endometriosis face a similar struggle. However, endometriosis has not gained mainstream recognition or understanding. Advocacy organizations are working to raise awareness of endometriosis, speed up diagnosis times, and increase research funding. In the U.S., the National Institutes of Health spends only $7 million annually on endometriosis research, despite the fact that it impacts over 6.5 million women. Endometriosis deserves the same level of recognition, understanding and research support that other similarly prevalent diseases receive. Like HIV/AIDS activists decades earlier, endometriosis advocates continue the fight against stigma and for equal treatment.

- **Endometriosis Often Overlooked and Misunderstood**

The symptoms of endometriosis are frequently dismissed or misattributed, leaving women struggling with severe pain and health issues that worsen over time without proper treatment. Similar to those living with HIV/AIDS in the 1980s, women with endometriosis today face stigma, lack of understanding, and limited options for medical care. They are frequently told that the pain is "normal" or that it is psychosomatic. It takes an average of 7 to 10 years for women to receive an endometriosis diagnosis after the onset of symptoms.

The gold standard for diagnosing endometriosis is laparoscopic surgery, but this procedure is often delayed or avoided due to costs, risks, and other factors. Medical management focuses on managing pain, slowing the growth of endometrial tissue, and improving quality of life. Options include pain medication, hormonal contraceptives, hormone therapy, pelvic floor therapy, and excision of endometrial lesions.

Like HIV/AIDS advocates of the past, the endometriosis community is working to raise awareness of the disease, reduce stigma, and push for more research and treatment options. By educating doctors, lawmakers, and the general public about endometriosis, patients and advocates hope to see reduced diagnosis times, better access to care, and new treatment options for managing symptoms or curing the disease. Though separated by decades, those living with endometriosis today face a strikingly similar fight as those who battled misunderstanding and discrimination during the rise of the HIV/AIDS epidemic. With time and effort, endometriosis may gain the same level of awareness and support in the medical community.

- **The Struggle to Access Treatment for Endometriosis**

Like those diagnosed with HIV/AIDS in the 1980s, women with endometriosis today face difficulties accessing medical care and effective treatment options.

Similar to HIV/AIDS in the 1980s, endometriosis is misunderstood and underfunded. Research on endometriosis receives a fraction of the funding of other diseases, and many doctors lack knowledge about diagnosis and treatment. Consequently, it takes an average of 8-12 years for women to receive an endometriosis diagnosis after the onset of symptoms.

Once diagnosed, treatment options are limited. Hormone therapy and pain medications may temporarily reduce symptoms but often cause undesirable side effects and do not treat the underlying disease. Laparoscopic excision surgery is considered the gold standard treatment, but few surgeons are skilled in the procedure, leading to long wait times.

Inadequate medical care and limited treatment choices force many women to cope with debilitating pain, infertility issues, and a decreased quality of life. Some turn to self-education and advocacy to raise awareness, push for policy changes, and help other women access better care. They share information about symptoms and treatment options, start support groups, and organize fundraising events. Their grassroots efforts are reminiscent of early HIV/AIDS activists working to accelerate research and improve patient care.

While medical understanding and options for both diseases have expanded over time, endometriosis still lacks many of the resources now available for HIV/AIDS management and prevention. However, the determination and activism of patients gives hope that in the coming decades, more women will receive treatment, funding, and scientific focus. Overall, endometriosis appears to be following a similar trajectory as HIV/AIDS in gaining recognition and resources, if at a slower pace. Continued advocacy and education efforts may help to speed up progress and improve outcomes.

- **The Need for More Research and Awareness of Endometriosis**

It affects approximately 176 million women worldwide, yet there is no known cure and limited treatment options available.

### The Need for More Research and Awareness

Endometriosis receives a small fraction of research funding compared to other diseases, despite the significant impact it has on women's health and quality of life. Increased funding is urgently needed to better understand the mechanisms behind the development and progression of the disease. Additional research on new treatment alternatives, improved screening techniques, and possible preventative measures could help the millions of women living with endometriosis.

Raising public awareness about endometriosis is also critical. Many women experience delays in diagnosis due to a lack of knowledge about the condition among healthcare professionals and the general public. Increased awareness and education can help address misconceptions, reduce stigma, and empower women to advocate for their health.

- Public health campaigns to educate women and girls about endometriosis symptoms and risk factors. This could help with early detection and diagnosis.

- Targeted education for healthcare professionals on accurately diagnosing and treating endometriosis. This includes general practitioners, gynecologists, and other specialists.

- Grassroots advocacy and support groups to raise funds for research, put pressure on policymakers, and share information within the endometriosis community.

- Celebrity endorsements and media coverage to bring mainstream attention to endometriosis as a significant women's health issue.

Decades after the emergence of HIV/AIDS, endometriosis remains misunderstood and underfunded. However, with more research and widespread awareness, there is hope that better treatments - and possibly even a cure - may be on the horizon. Overall, a multi-pronged approach across public, private, and non-profit sectors is needed to drive progress for this chronic and debilitating disease. The women living with endometriosis deserve nothing less.

- **HIV/AIDS Activists Paved the Way for the Endometriosis Community**

The HIV/AIDS epidemic in the 1980s faced many of the same challenges that the endometriosis community faces today. Activists for both causes have had to fight to raise awareness, reduce stigma, and gain recognition and funding.

In the early days of the HIV/AIDS epidemic, the medical community struggled to understand the new disease. Lack of knowledge and stigma caused many in the public and private sectors to avoid addressing the crisis. Activists worked tirelessly to raise awareness, educate policymakers, and demand funding and research. Similarly, endometriosis has been misunderstood and stigmatized due to lack of research and education. The endometriosis community has had to advocate to raise awareness, gain recognition and increase research on symptoms, diagnosis, and treatment.

For those with HIV/AIDS, discrimination and stigma were major obstacles. Many faced ostracization due to myths about transmission and high-risk groups. Endometriosis also carries a stigma due to its relation to menstruation and reproduction. Many with endometriosis face discrimination in education and the workplace due to debilitating symptoms and time off needed for treatment. Both groups have fought against prejudice and misconceptions to gain acceptance and support.

In the 1980s, HIV/AIDS activists demanded funding and research to better understand the disease and develop effective treatments. The endometriosis community has similarly had to advocate for research funding to improve diagnosis, find alternative treatments, and work toward a cure. After decades of effort, activists for both causes have made progress but still have further to go.

The battles fought by HIV/AIDS activists in the 1980s helped pave the way for disease advocacy and support groups of all kinds, including the endometriosis community. By raising their voices against stigma and demanding change, they helped legitimize the experience of patients and give advocacy efforts a model to follow. Though separated by decades, the challenges faced in the fight against HIV/AIDS and endometriosis are more alike than different. Both groups give a face to misunderstood medical issues and work to build a more just and inclusive society.

Thirty years separate the emergence of HIV/AIDS and the rise of advocacy for endometriosis, yet the struggles faced by both groups share striking similarities. Discrimination, lack of education, and insufficient funding have made progress agonizingly slow for each medical issue. However, through the tireless efforts of activists, scientists, and those personally impacted, there is hope on the horizon. Continued support of research and open conversations about these health conditions can chip away at stigma, improve treatments, and save lives. No one should have to suffer in silence or fight alone against a disease that threatens their well-being and quality of life. Though separated by time, HIV/AIDS activists of the past and endometriosis advocates of today are united in their mission to overcome. The future is brighter because of the battles they've chosen to wage together.

# 17

## ENDOMETRIOSIS: MISUNDERSTOOD, MISTREATED, MARGINALIZED

Endometriosis requires the same advocacy and awareness efforts that have benefited other diseases. It's time we come together to demand improved diagnostic techniques, more effective treatments, and destigmatize this debilitating condition so that women no longer feel isolated in their suffering. No woman should have to fight to have her pain recognized and treated. Together, we can bring endometriosis out of the shadows and inspire action through education and open discussion. The status quo is unacceptable, and women deserve so much better.

**Why Endometriosis Is So Often Misdiagnosed**

There are several reasons why endometriosis continues to elude medical professionals:

Symptoms are often mistaken for normal menstrual pain. Pelvic pain, painful intercourse, painful urination during menses, and gastrointestinal issues are frequently misinterpreted as typical period problems. In reality, they can indicate the presence of endometrial tissue outside the uterus.

Pelvic exams and ultrasounds may appear normal. Endometriosis cannot be detected through routine gynecological exams or standard imaging. Laparoscopic surgery is required for an accurate diagnosis, but due to cost and risk, doctors often try other options first.

Menstruation is stigmatized. Discussing menstrual health issues can be uncomfortable for patients and doctors alike, allowing manageable symptoms to progress into chronic pain before seeking answers.

Research and education are lacking. The complex mechanisms behind endometriosis development and progression are not fully understood. More research is urgently needed to find non-invasive, affordable diagnostic tools as well as alternative treatments beyond surgery and hormones.

Doctors are not properly trained. Most physicians receive little education about endometriosis, leading to misdiagnosis and inadequate treatment. Patients often suffer for years before finding an endometriosis specialist. Endometriosis may be a common disease, but it remains misunderstood, mistreated, and marginalized. Through advocacy, activism, and medical advancement, there is hope for earlier diagnosis, better care, and ultimately, a cure.

Living with endometriosis often comes with an emotional toll that is not fully understood or acknowledged. The chronic pain, fatigue, and other debilitating symptoms significantly impact your quality of life and mental health. Endometriosis is an invisible illness, meaning that the internal damage and suffering are not outwardly apparent. This can lead to feelings of isolation and lack of support. The pain and other symptoms are very real but because they are not "seen," they are often dismissed or diminished by others. Many with endometriosis report being told their pain is "normal" or that they are exaggerating or being overdramatic. This lack of validation and empathy only serves to intensify the emotional suffering.

Endometriosis involves the growth of endometrial tissue outside of the uterus. This abnormal cell growth leads to a loss of control over your own body and bodily functions. You may experience pain, bleeding, or other symptoms without warning that disrupt your daily activities and plans. This loss of control and unpredictability causes significant distress, anxiety, and depression in many with the condition.

In addition to lack of visibility, endometriosis is often misunderstood and mistreated due to gender bias in medicine. Many report struggling to be heard, believed, and taken seriously by doctors when describing their pain and symptoms. They face delayed diagnosis and inappropriate or ineffective treatments as a result. The need to advocate strongly for yourself to get proper diagnosis and care only adds to the emotional labor of this condition. Overall, the psychological impact of endometriosis is substantial and complex, going far beyond the physical symptoms alone. Recognition, validation, and support are urgently needed. With greater understanding and advocacy, the emotional suffering for those with endometriosis can be reduced.

There are limited treatment options for endometriosis, and none provide a cure. Hormonal contraceptives and pain medications only provide temporary relief from symptoms. Surgery to remove endometrial tissue is often ineffective, as the tissue frequently grows back. The inability of modern medicine to develop curative or long-term treatments for such a common disease is unacceptable and reflects the historical tendency to dismiss women's pain. Additional research funding and efforts are urgently needed.

Endometriosis is stigmatized due to its association with menstruation, a natural bodily process that is still taboo to discuss openly in many cultures. As a result, many women suffer in silence, unaware that their painful periods are not normal and that treatment options exist. Doctors frequently dismiss or misdiagnose women's reports of severe menstrual pain. When a diagnosis of endometriosis is made, women are often told that pain is simply a part of being a woman or that pregnancy will cure the condition. These biased attitudes contribute to the marginalization of people with endometriosis.

Despite affecting approximately 176 million women worldwide, endometriosis remains poorly understood and funded. There are few public awareness campaigns for endometriosis compared to other medical conditions that affect a similar number of people. Robust advocacy and education efforts are needed to increase research funding, improve diagnostic rates, and provide better support for those living with endometriosis. By raising awareness of endometriosis as a serious chronic illness, we can help end the marginalization of those who suffer from it.

The lack of effective treatments, pervasive social stigma, and inadequate advocacy and awareness surrounding endometriosis all contribute to its marginalized status. Concerted efforts across healthcare, research, and advocacy sectors are urgently needed to bring endometriosis into the mainstream, reduce suffering, and improve quality of life for millions of women.

Oral contraceptives and hormonal IUDs are commonly prescribed to help reduce pain from endometriosis. However, they do not eradicate endometrial lesions and symptoms typically return once treatment is stopped. These medications also do not work for all individuals and can cause undesirable side effects like mood changes, weight gain, and loss of libido.

Over the counter and prescription pain relievers may be used to manage endometriosis discomfort.

Similar to hormonal treatments, these only provide temporary relief from symptoms. Long-term use or high doses of painkillers can also lead to dependence and damage internal organs.

Laparoscopic surgery is often performed to remove visible endometrial tissue growths. While surgery may provide relief from symptoms for a period of months or years, there is a high chance of recurrence as microscopic lesions are often left behind or new growths form. Repeat surgeries also increase health risks and the potential for surgical complications.

Some individuals have found relief from alternative treatments like acupuncture, massage therapy, dietary changes, and herbal medicine. However, there is little scientific evidence to support the effectiveness of most alternative therapies for endometriosis. They may provide a placebo effect or temporary reduction in symptoms for some but are unlikely to treat the underlying disease. For myself, this is the route I take, and this is my way of making life more manageable for myself.

The current medical options for managing endometriosis are imperfect and inadequate. More research is desperately needed to develop treatments that can eliminate lesions, reduce inflammation, prevent recurrence, and ultimately cure this debilitating disease. Until that time, many endometriosis sufferers will continue to face a life of chronic pain and compromised quality of life.

Building a community of advocates is crucial to raising awareness and improving treatments for endometriosis. By banding together, individuals can apply pressure to increase research funding, improve access to care, and reduce stigma. At the beginning of this book, you can find a link to a group we have created for you all to join and help us spread awareness and build a community.

The first step is educating people about endometriosis - what it is, how it impacts those affected, available treatments (or lack thereof), and obstacles faced. Explain that endometriosis occurs when tissue similar to the lining of the uterus grows outside of the uterus, causing pain, infertility, and other issues. Spread awareness that there is no cure and limited treatment options. Share statistics, like the average 7–12-year delay in diagnosis, to demonstrate the need for earlier detection and more research.

Connect with others in the endometriosis community to share experiences, advice, and support. Look for local support groups, online forums, Facebook groups, and nonprofits like the Endometriosis Association and the Endometriosis Foundation of America. Getting involved in the broader community helps reduce feelings of isolation and gives a platform to advocate for change.

There are many ways individuals can take action to advance the cause. Write to representatives in Congress and healthcare organizations to push for more research funding and improved standards of care. Sign petitions calling for recognition of endometriosis as a chronic illness. Participate in awareness campaigns like EndoMarch to spread information. Share personal experiences on social media using hashtags like #EndoAwareness, #WeEndoWarriors, and #EndoMarch to put a human face on the disease. Join our support and educational community at:

https://endo-warriors-collective.mn.co/

Progress will require persistent and vocal advocacy. Stay up to date with the latest research studies, treatments in development, and policy changes that could impact those with endometriosis. Continue applying pressure and making noise to keep endometriosis in the spotlight. Significant improvements may take years, but by banding together as a community, there is hope for accelerating diagnosis, expanding treatment options, and ultimately finding a cure. Collective action can drive real change.

Coping with endometriosis day-to-day can be challenging, but there are some practical tips to help manage pain and symptoms:

*Track your symptoms!*

Keeping a symptom journal or calendar can help identify patterns in pain, bleeding, and hormonal changes. Note the severity, duration, and possible triggers of symptoms each day. Look for links between your cycle, diet, exercise, stress levels, and flare-ups.

Spotting these connections will allow you to make lifestyle changes and better predict (and hopefully prevent) episodes of severe pain.

### *Practice self-care*

Engage in regular self-care to help reduce stress and ease symptoms. Get enough sleep, limit alcohol and caffeine, exercise gently, and eat an anti-inflammatory diet high in fresh fruits and vegetables, whole grains, and lean protein. Some women find relief from acupuncture, massage therapy, mindfulness exercises like meditation or yoga. Don't forget to schedule in downtime to rest when you need it.

### *Try Herbal Approaches*

Look into herbal medicine, herbology has been around for more than a millennia and is what majority of our medications today are derived from. I found that starting over at the basics has really helped me a lot. We will be releasing another book with such details for you all to check out, but you really can do your own research and find most of what you need in your own yards. We will also be providing herbal medicine classes in the

Endo Warriors Collective (https://endo-warriors-collective.mn.co/).

## *Try Apple Cider Vinegar and Dietary Changes*

Here again these are methods I personally use. ACV is alkaline and suffocates any harmful substances in your body. There for it has the ability to suffocate endometriosis within the proper PH levels. More information on the benefits of AVC can be found most anywhere with a simple google search or even in holistic books. I have also found that dropping most if not all acidic foods and drinks has helped me get some life back. I feel much better overall and the number of flare-ups I experience monthly has greatly decreased. When I do get off diet, I almost immediately feel awful, and I experience a flair up the following week.

## *Use over the counter medications*

For pain management, start with mild over-the-counter medications like ibuprofen, naproxen, or acetaminophen. Apply heating pads to sore areas, use a TENS unit, or get prescription pain medication from your doctor if needed. Hormonal birth control like contraceptive pills can also help reduce pain and the heaviness of periods. Always follow the instructions and don't take these medications long-term unless directed to do so by your physician.

### *Talk to your doctor about treatment options!*

Discuss medical and surgical options for managing endometriosis with your gynecologist. Prescription hormonal therapies like GnRH agonists may help slow the growth of lesions and reduce symptoms. For severe cases, laparoscopic excision surgery to remove lesions and scar tissue can provide longer lasting relief when performed by a specialist. Don't lose hope - new treatment options are on the horizon. We understand this is the very last thing any of us want to do after years of being thrown aside and ignored. Keep in mind there is hope and not all doctors are the same. Keep fighting, keep looking.

Living with endometriosis often means adapting your self-care routine and treatment options over time. But by tracking your symptoms, reducing stress, managing pain, and working closely with your doctor, you can find an approach that helps you cope from day to day and continue living life fully despite the challenges of this condition. Staying proactive and maintaining a positive attitude will serve you well in your journey towards symptom relief and empowerment.

Endometriosis continues to be a puzzling health issue that requires more research and advocacy to improve diagnosis, treatment, and quality of life for those affected. Through education and open conversation, we can work to eliminate the stigma surrounding this chronic and often debilitating disease.

As someone living with endometriosis, you know this disease is poorly understood and treated. You've experienced firsthand the lack of effective treatments, the stigma surrounding "women's problems", and the need for more advocacy and awareness. Though endometriosis affects 1 in 10 women, research on this disease receives a fraction of the funding of other conditions. You deserve better.

You are not alone in this fight. By speaking up about your experiences, participating in surveys and studies, and supporting advocacy organizations pushing for more research funding and physician education, together we can drive real change. Endometriosis may be incurable today, but through collective action we can work to improve diagnosis, develop new treatments, and gain mainstream recognition of this debilitating disease. Staying silent will only allow the status quo to persist. Raise your voice – it is time endometriosis becomes a health priority. Together, we have the power to make that happen.

# 18

# FIGHTING THE GOOD FIGHT: APPLYING HIV/AIDS ADVOCACY TACTICS TO ENDOMETRIOSIS

As an endometriosis sufferer, you know the frustration of this invisible disease. However, we can take lessons from successful health advocacy campaigns and apply them to endometriosis. The HIV/AIDS movement revolutionized how diseases are researched and treated. By adopting similar advocacy tactics, we can bring endometriosis out of the shadows.

We must speak up to spread awareness, share our stories to build empathy, and lobby policymakers for funding and support. Although endometriosis is a different disease, HIV/AIDS advocates paved the way by proving patient voices have power. Together, we can follow their lead. We can educate doctors and the public, tackle stigma, and campaign for research. Every voice matters in creating change.

Staying silent won't make endometriosis go away. But raising our voices just might gain us ground in finding better treatments and a cure. The advocacy fight ahead won't be easy, but for the chance to gain understanding and relief, it's a fight worth having. After years of struggling in secret, we owe it to ourselves and others to make some noise. The time for action is now. Our advocacy efforts can make all the difference in this good fight.

In the early days of the HIV/AIDS epidemic, stigma and misinformation were rampant. Marginalized groups disproportionately affected faced discrimination and prejudice, while lack of education left everyone at risk.

To combat this, activists organized to raise awareness and advocate for change. They lobbied governments to increase funding for research and treatment. They launched public education campaigns to spread facts about transmission and prevention. They fought for policies protecting the rights of those living with HIV/AIDS.

Public figures came out about their HIV status, humanizing the disease. TV shows featured characters with HIV, showing they could live full lives with proper treatment. Activists gave speeches, organizing fundraising and awareness events. They made HIV/AIDS impossible to ignore, building empathy and understanding.

Activists formed coalitions across groups, recognizing shared interests. The LGBTQ community and public health organizations worked together. Faith leaders and activists partnered to reach communities. These alliances strengthened advocacy efforts through collaboration.

Lawmakers were lobbied to prohibit discrimination against those with HIV/AIDS and fund research. The Ryan White Comprehensive AIDS Resources Emergency (CARE) Act provided treatment for low-income and uninsured patients. Activists pushed for accelerated approval of life-saving drugs. With perseverance, they changed laws and influenced budget priorities.

The HIV/AIDS movement offers a blueprint for advocacy around stigmatized health issues. By raising public awareness, forging alliances, and lobbying for policy changes, activists helped turn the tide against misinformation and discrimination. Applying similar tactics, the endometriosis community can make progress toward better understanding, treatment, and support. But first we must come together, share our stories, and speak up for change.

To enact real change, endometriosis advocates must follow the successful tactics used by HIV/AIDS activists. HIV/AIDS advocates were able to:

Challenge stigma and misconceptions about the disease. They launched public awareness campaigns to educate people about how HIV/AIDS is transmitted and addressed myths about who it affects. Endometriosis advocates need to challenge the notion that it only impacts fertility or is not a real medical condition.

Put pressure on policymakers and demand government action. HIV/AIDS activists lobbied governments to increase research funding and make new treatments available. Similarly, endometriosis advocates must call on policymakers to increase funding for research into the causes and better treatment options for this chronic condition.

Build coalitions and alliances. HIV/AIDS activists were able to unite many groups under a common goal. Endometriosis advocates should work to build coalitions with women's health groups, chronic pain organizations and healthcare professionals to strengthen their efforts.

Insist on patient involvement in decision making. HIV/AIDS activists demanded to be included in the process for developing new treatments and shaping policies. Endometriosis advocates need to push for more patient representation on advisory boards and policy committees to ensure the patient perspective is considered.

By coming together, raising awareness, and advocating for political and policy changes, endometriosis activists can achieve similar successes as HIV/AIDS advocates before them. With perseverance and unity, real progress can be made for the millions of women living with this disease. The fight will be difficult but following the model of determined and committed advocacy groups can lead to better outcomes, just as it did for those with HIV/AIDS.

There are several parallels that can be drawn between the HIV/AIDS epidemic and endometriosis that advocacy groups can utilize to raise awareness and push for better treatment and research.

Similar to how HIV/AIDS was once considered a "gay disease," endometriosis is frequently mischaracterized as solely a "women's disease." This contributes to the lack of research and funding, as well as stigma surrounding the condition. Advocacy groups should work to reframe endometriosis as a disease that affects people of all genders in order to gain broader support and understanding.

Both HIV/AIDS and endometriosis are chronic, incurable conditions that significantly impact quality of life. People living with endometriosis frequently face pain, infertility, loss of work, and difficulty with daily activities, similar to the way those with HIV/AIDS experience ongoing health issues and disability. By framing endometriosis as a life-altering disease rather than a normal part of menstruation, advocacy groups can better convey the seriousness of this condition to healthcare professionals, policymakers, and the public.

There are also parallels in the journey to diagnosis and effective treatment for those with endometriosis and HIV/AIDS. It often takes years of advocating for oneself to receive an accurate diagnosis and find a treatment plan that provides relief from symptoms. Unfortunately, the medical system continues to fail many with these diseases. Advocacy groups should put pressure on physicians and policymakers to improve diagnosis, treatment, and management of endometriosis to prevent unnecessary suffering.

The HIV/AIDS epidemic has shown us that patient advocacy and activism can drive critical changes. By drawing parallels between these diseases and utilizing proven advocacy tactics, the endometriosis community can work to build awareness, increase funding for research and gain better access to medical care. With a unified voice, people of all genders affected by endometriosis can fight for understanding, empowerment, and hope.

## Lesson 1: Educate the Public and Fight Misinformation

To effectively advocate for increased research and improved treatment of endometriosis, educating the public and healthcare professionals about the disease is essential. Endometriosis remains poorly understood, even in the medical community, leading to delayed diagnosis and misinformation.

### Spreading Awareness

The first step is raising public awareness about endometriosis symptoms and impacts. Many people still believe endometriosis is "just bad cramps," when in reality it can be an excruciating and debilitating disease. Educating people about the range of symptoms, like chronic pelvic pain, painful intercourse, and infertility, helps build understanding. Developing a strong online presence through social media campaigns, podcasts, news media, and blog posts is key. Creating a hashtag, like #EndoAware, #WeEndoWarriors, or #EndoTruth, gives people a way to share stories and start conversations.

## Correcting Myths

There are many myths about endometriosis that stand in the way of progress. It is not true that endometriosis only impacts women in their 30s and 40s, that hysterectomy cures it, that it cannot impact fertility, or that birth control pills effectively manage symptoms for most women. Correcting these myths and highlighting facts about endometriosis, especially among healthcare providers, is vital. Providing continuing medical education on diagnosis and treatment can help reduce delays and misdiagnoses.

## Framing the Issue

How endometriosis is framed also matters. Rather than portraying it solely as a "women's health" issue, endometriosis should be recognized as a public health issue that impacts families, relationships, and society. Framing it this way helps build understanding of the far-reaching impacts and the need for improved care and resources. The economic costs of endometriosis on individuals and society are substantial, another reason this framing is important.

Using tactics that worked for HIV/AIDS advocacy, like public education campaigns, myth-busting, and strategic framing of the issue, can be effective for endometriosis. Spreading awareness, promoting understanding, and advocating for change has the power to transform outcomes and reduce suffering for millions of women around the world.

**Lesson 2: Advocate for More Research Funding**

To advocate effectively for increased research funding, activists must make a compelling case for why more resources are urgently needed. For endometriosis, building a strong rationale involves:

**Demonstrating the Scale of the Problem**

Endometriosis impacts roughly 176 million women worldwide, according to the World Endometriosis Society, yet it receives a fraction of the research funding of other similarly prevalent diseases. Activists must publicize statistics on the prevalence, health impacts, and economic costs of endometriosis to show policymakers why more research is vital to public health.

### Highlighting the Lack of Treatment Options

There are currently no cures for endometriosis, only treatments that temporarily relieve symptoms. Activists should emphasize the limited treatment choices available, and the risks associated with existing options like hormonal therapies. More research is needed to develop safer, more effective interventions.

### Identifying Knowledge Gaps

While endometriosis has been recognized as a disease for over a century, there are still many unanswered questions about its causes, progression, and optimal management. Activists should pinpoint specific areas where more research is needed, such as the role of genetics and the environment, novel treatment targets, and improved surgical techniques. Closing these knowledge gaps could transform care for those living with this enigmatic condition.

### Building Public Support

To spur political will for change, activists must raise awareness of endometriosis and build grassroots support for the cause. By sharing personal stories of living with endometriosis and organizing community events, activists can help the public understand the realities of this disease and the need to prioritize research funding. With enough voices speaking out, policymakers will have to listen and take action.

By making a compelling case for the scale, impacts and knowledge gaps of endometriosis, and rallying public support, activists can apply powerful advocacy strategies that drove progress against HIV/AIDS to push for greatly increased research funding. Significant investments in research are urgently needed to improve understanding of this disease and develop better solutions for the millions affected worldwide.

## Lesson 3: Push for Compassionate, Patient-Cantered Care

To improve care for endometriosis patients, advocacy groups should push healthcare systems and providers to adopt a compassionate, patient-centred model of care.

### Listen to Patients

Healthcare providers should make the effort to understand patients' experiences and perspectives. Patients often report feeling unheard or dismissed, with their symptoms and concerns attributed to normal menstruation or psychological issues.

Providers should take the time to listen without judgment and validate patients' experiences. Asking open-ended questions about symptoms, medical history, challenges, and the impact on quality of life can help build understanding and guide diagnosis and treatment.

**Provide Holistic Support**

Endometriosis frequently causes chronic pain, infertility, and other issues that significantly impact wellbeing. However, care is often focused narrowly on physical symptoms. A holistic, integrated approach addresses psychological, emotional, and social challenges in addition to medical needs.

**This could include:**

- Referrals to therapists and support groups

- Discussing the emotional impact of infertility or hysterectomy

- Connecting patients with advocacy organizations for education and community

- Recommending alternative therapies like acupuncture, massage, or yoga to improve quality of life in a safe, monitored way.

- Share Decision Making

Providers should involve patients in developing treatment plans, explaining options and collaborating on the best course of action based on priorities and values. This empowers patients and leads to plans that address their unique situation and needs.

Making the effort to show compassion, listen without judgment and share decision making can vastly improve the care experience for endometriosis patients. Healthcare systems and providers should make these patient-centered practices a priority, with the goal of not just treating symptoms but supporting overall health and wellbeing. By advocating for this model of care, endometriosis organizations can push for sustainable change that benefits members and the broader community.

## Lesson 4: Build Community and Support Systems

To effectively advocate for those with endometriosis, it is crucial to build community support systems. By fostering connections between individuals impacted by the disease, advocacy organizations can enhance their influence and better achieve their goals.

### Establish Local Support Groups

Local support groups provide a way for those with endometriosis to find companionship and exchange information. Organizations should work to establish support groups in communities nationwide. These groups can meet in person or online to discuss experiences with the disease, recommend doctors and treatments, and provide empathy. Over time, support group members may become actively involved in broader advocacy efforts. Join us at https://endo-warriors-collective.mn.co/.

### Develop Online Forums

In addition to local groups, online forums and message boards give those with endometriosis a way to connect on a larger scale. Advocacy organizations should create and promote moderated forums where individuals can post questions, share stories, and offer advice. These online communities can help endometriosis patients feel less alone in their experience. They also provide a platform to discuss advocacy priorities and organize around specific campaigns.

### Build Partnerships

To maximize impact, endometriosis advocacy organizations should pursue strategic partnerships with other nonprofits, healthcare providers, and companies. Collaboration with women's health organizations, chronic illness alliances, and pain management groups can help raise awareness of endometriosis as a serious disease. Partnerships with clinics, hospitals, and medical practices will improve patient support and access to knowledgeable doctors. Corporate alliances may provide financial backing for advocacy programs as part of their social responsibility efforts.

### Train Ambassadors

Selecting and training a team of ambassadors to represent the endometriosis community is an effective way to spread awareness and advance advocacy goals. Ambassadors can share their experiences through public speaking events, media opportunities, and community outreach. They act as the "face" of the advocacy organization and help put a human story behind the mission. With proper training and support, ambassadors become empowered to lobby lawmakers, promote campaigns, and champion policy changes on behalf of those impacted by endometriosis.

Building a network of support and empowering individuals to take action is key to creating an influential advocacy movement. By following the examples of successful campaigns like HIV/AIDS advocacy, endometriosis organizations can strengthen their base, raise their collective voice, and work toward better health outcomes for all.

**Lesson 5: Lobby for Legislative Changes**

To enact meaningful legislative changes, advocates must lobby elected officials and policymakers. Some effective tactics include:

## Educate Legislators About the Issue

Endometriosis advocates should provide legislators and their staff with educational materials explaining the disease, its prevalence and impact. Explain that endometriosis affects over 11% of women worldwide, causing severe pain, infertility, and decreased quality of life.

## Share Personal Stories

Personal stories from constituents who live with endometriosis are extremely compelling and help put a human face on the issue. Meet with legislators and share how endometriosis has affected your health, relationships, career, and daily activities. Explain specific ways that policy changes could help improve your situation.

## Build Grassroots Support

Grassroots advocacy campaigns that demonstrate substantial constituent support are persuasive to lawmakers. Endometriosis organizations should mobilize supporters to call, write and meet with their elected officials asking them to take action on key legislative priorities. Lawmakers want to support issues their constituents care about.

### Propose Specific Policy Solutions

In addition to describing the problem, advocates must propose concrete policy solutions and ask lawmakers to take specific actions. For endometriosis, this could include increased research funding, improved insurance coverage for diagnosis and treatment, and designated women's health coordinators in federal agencies. Provide lawmakers with draft bill language they can introduce.

### Work Across the Aisle

Effective advocacy requires working with lawmakers from both political parties. While some public health issues become politicized, endometriosis is a bipartisan women's health concern. Build relationships and work with both Democratic and Republican officials to find common ground and make incremental progress. Compromise and willingness to accept less than ideal solutions are often needed to achieve real policy changes.

Continual education, personal stories, grassroots mobilization and proposing specific policy solutions are proven techniques that endometriosis advocates can apply to successfully lobby for legislative progress. Building bipartisan support and willingness to compromise are also key. By working together across party lines, the endometriosis community can achieve meaningful policy changes to drive research, improve care and support those living with this disease.

## Turning Knowledge into Action: What You Can Do for Endometriosis Advocacy

Knowing the challenges endometriosis presents is not enough. For real change to happen, you must take action. Here are a few ways you can advocate for the endometriosis community:

### Contact Your Elected Officials

Reach out to your representatives in Congress and ask them to support legislation like the Endometriosis Health and Education Act. Explain how endometriosis impacts you or your loved one's life and health. Share your story—it will make a difference.

## Support Endometriosis Organizations

Nonprofits like the Endometriosis Foundation of America, the Endometriosis Association, and local support groups need your help to raise awareness and fund research. Donate your time by volunteering or money by becoming a member. Work with them on initiatives and attend or help organize local events.

## Share Your Experience

Speak up about living with endometriosis. Start conversations, especially with friends and family, to spread understanding. Share articles and information on social media. Talk about it on your blog or podcast. The more people understand endometriosis, the less stigmatized and isolated those with the disease will feel.

## Participate in Clinical Trials

New treatments can only be approved if there are participants in clinical trials to test them. Search for endometriosis-related trials on ClinicalTrials.gov and enroll if you qualify. Even if you receive a placebo, you are advancing research that could help future generations.

**Make Lifestyle Changes**

Certain lifestyle adjustments may help reduce endometriosis symptoms and pain. A balanced diet low in red meat and high in fresh fruits and vegetables, exercise like yoga or walking, limiting alcohol, and quitting smoking are all steps in the right direction. While not a cure, a healthy lifestyle can enhance your wellbeing. Making these changes also shows solidarity with others in the endometriosis community working to improve their lives in face of this chronic illness.

The key is to start where you are and do what you can. Every action makes a difference in creating change and moving closer to better outcomes, less suffering, and hope for the over 176 million women worldwide with endometriosis. Together, we can turn knowledge into action.

You now have a blueprint for advocating for increased awareness and funding for endometriosis. By following the tactics that proved successful for HIV/AIDS advocates, you can help enact real change. Educate the public and key stakeholders. Build alliances and coalitions to strengthen your voice. Put pressure on policymakers and companies through organized campaigns. Share stories to give endometriosis a human face. The challenges may seem daunting, but taking action together, progress can be made. Though the road ahead is long, stay determined and focused on the destination of improved treatment, greater understanding, and ultimately, a cure. The lessons of the past can guide us.

# PART 5

## LACK OF KNOWLEDGE AND AWARNESS

# 19

## THE SILENT SUFFERING: ENDOMETRIOSIS AWARENESS AND THE URGENT NEED FOR EDUCATION

# The Agonizing Reality of Living with Endometriosis

Living with endometriosis is agonizing, to say the least. The pain is relentless - sharp stabs, dull aches, cramping that leaves you breathless. It permeates every aspect of your life, making even simple tasks excruciating. There is no escaping it.

You desperately seek relief, trying every over-the-counter and prescription painkiller. Some days you can't get out of bed. Calling in sick to work or school again, cancelling plans with friends, missing out on life - it becomes your normal.

Doctors often dismiss your symptoms as "just cramps" or exaggeration. It can take years of suffering before receiving an accurate diagnosis. And even after the diagnosis, treatment options are limited. Hormone therapy may provide temporary relief, but the endo frequently returns. Repeated surgeries have risks, and the endo can recur again.

Living with an invisible yet debilitating disease like endometriosis leads to feelings of isolation, anxiety, and depression. Your relationships, career and self-esteem suffer. Simple things others take for granted, like going to the movies or exercising, require meticulous planning around pain and fatigue.

Endometriosis awareness is urgently needed. This disease deserves more research funding and attention, and healthcare providers require better education to reduce diagnosis and treatment delays. Women need more support and validation of their experience. Although there is no cure yet, with increased knowledge there is hope for improved management options so fewer have to endure years of silent suffering.

## Widespread Misconceptions About Endometriosis

Endometriosis is shrouded in widespread misconceptions that lead to the suffering of millions of women.

### The Myth of "Normal" Menstrual Pain

Too many women are told that severe pain during menstruation is "normal" or "just part of being a woman." The truth is painful periods can be a sign that something's wrong. If your cramps regularly disrupt your life, don't brush them off - talk to your doctor. Endometriosis could be the cause of your suffering.

**Infertility is Not Always a Consequence**

While endometriosis can contribute to infertility in some cases, many women with endometriosis are still able to get pregnant. The severity and location of endometrial lesions as well as a woman's age all play a role in fertility. With treatment, the chances of natural conception and success with assisted reproductive technologies are good for many endometriosis patients.

**Hysterectomy is Not the Only Option**

A hysterectomy, or removal of the uterus, is often mistakenly viewed as a "cure" for endometriosis. But endometrial tissue can grow on other pelvic organs, so a hysterectomy alone may not eliminate pain and symptoms. There are now many minimally invasive treatment options for endometriosis that can provide relief while preserving fertility. A hysterectomy should only be considered as a last resort for severe, persistent cases that do not respond to other therapies.

Through education and advocacy, we can spread awareness about this "silent" disease and correct long-held misbeliefs. Endometriosis patients deserve understanding, compassion, and healthcare that meets their needs. Together, we can make a difference.

## Improving Endometriosis Care Through Education and Awareness

Endometriosis remains underdiagnosed and poorly understood by many in the general public and even within the healthcare community. This lack of awareness and education surrounding the condition contributes greatly to the suffering of those affected.

### Improving Diagnosis and Treatment

Endometriosis care starts with equipping doctors and nurses with the knowledge to recognize signs and symptoms, enabling faster diagnosis and treatment. Too often, women endure months or even years of chronic pelvic pain and other symptoms before receiving an endometriosis diagnosis. Education on the latest treatment options for doctors can also help patients find relief.

Provide physicians and nurses with targeted education on identifying endometriosis symptoms.

Increase awareness of the latest treatments like excision surgery and hormonal therapies that may offer improved outcomes.

Make educational resources on endometriosis diagnosis and management freely available for healthcare professionals.

### Educating and Empowering Patients

Arming women with knowledge about endometriosis is key. When patients understand their condition better, they can advocate for themselves to get the care they need. Resources should aim to:

Explain the symptoms, causes, and treatment options for endometriosis in an easy-to-understand way.

Highlight the importance of early diagnosis and finding an endometriosis specialist.

Share stories from other women with endometriosis to build understanding and solidarity.

Provide guidance on managing pain, fatigue, and other symptoms to improve quality of life.

Through education and improved awareness, endometriosis care can be transformed. Equipping doctors and empowering patients with knowledge is the first step to reducing suffering and ensuring better outcomes for all those affected. By working together, we can make a difference.

So don't suffer in silence. Speak up and spread the word. Endometriosis affects approximately 176 million women worldwide - that's a lot of people living with pain every day of their lives. There is still no known cure, but with increased awareness and education comes faster diagnosis, improved treatment options and better quality of life. You have the power to change that by sharing this information with your friends, family, coworkers, and doctors. Together, we can raise our voices to put endometriosis in the spotlight. Talk about it, ask questions and support organizations promoting research and advocacy. You are not alone, and there is hope. Every small act of understanding and compassion gets us one step closer to a world without endometriosis. You can be a part of the movement that makes that happen.

# 20

## LOST YEARS OF PAIN: THE LASTING IMPACT OF DELAYED ENDOMETRIOSIS DIAGNOSIS

For too many with endometriosis, diagnosis takes over 7 years. Valuable time is lost to a lack of knowledge and understanding of this painful disorder. Time lost to inadequate support and treatment. Time no one can give back. But there is hope - through advocacy, education and research, the future for endometriosis diagnosis and care is changing. The lost years of pain may soon be a thing of the past.

## The Agony of Undiagnosed Endometriosis

The years of pain before diagnosis are some of the darkest for women with endometriosis. Without a name for the agony, there seems no end in sight. Doctors frequently dismiss or misdiagnose symptoms, leaving women feeling hopeless and alone.

By the time you receive an accurate diagnosis, the disease may have progressed significantly. Endometrial lesions or cysts, known as endometriomas, can form and spread to other areas like the bowels or bladder. Growths may fuse organs together or form scar tissue. This can lead to a host of complications like infertility, increased pain, and a higher risk of hysterectomy.

The psychological toll is also immense. Living with chronic pain and no answers can lead to depression, anxiety, feelings of isolation, and even post-traumatic stress disorder. Many women report that doctors made them feel like the pain was "all in their head" or that they had a low pain tolerance. This compounds an already difficult situation, damaging self-esteem, and the ability to advocate for proper care.

After diagnosis, women often look back with sorrow at the years lost to suffering in silence. But with diagnosis comes validation, community support, and treatment options to reclaim life from the clutches of this insidious disease. While the road ahead may still be long, at last there are answers and hope for a pain-free future.

## How Lack of Awareness Delays Diagnosis and Treatment

When endometriosis is misdiagnosed or undiagnosed for years, the physical and emotional damage can be devastating. By the time you finally get the correct diagnosis, you've often already lost years of your life to unexplained pelvic pain and heavy periods.

Not knowing what's wrong with your own body is a frightening experience. Doctors may dismiss your symptoms as "normal" or blame them on other issues like irritable bowel syndrome. This lack of awareness and understanding about endometriosis among physicians delays diagnosis and access to treatment.

By the time endometriosis is detected, adhesions and scar tissue have usually already formed and spread within the pelvis. This can lead to infertility, bowel or bladder problems, and impaired quality of life. Treatment then becomes more complicated, and a hysterectomy is more likely to be recommended.

Living with undiagnosed endometriosis also takes a major psychological toll. When your pain is repeatedly dismissed, you start to doubt yourself and lose hope. Feelings of isolation and even depression are common. Connecting with support groups can help combat this, but without a diagnosis, many don't know where to turn.

Increased awareness about endometriosis among doctors and the public is urgently needed. Earlier diagnosis and treatment can prevent years of suffering and loss. Ongoing support and understanding would transform the lives of the millions of women with this disease. Together, we can work to make endometriosis more visible and help those affected get their lives back.

## The Ripple Effects of Late Diagnosis on Women's Lives

When endometriosis goes undiagnosed for years, it can have far-reaching effects on all areas of a woman's life. By the time you get a diagnosis, the disease may have already caused severe damage.

The pain and discomfort from endometriosis can make it difficult to work, attend school, spend time with loved ones, or engage in physical activities. You may have missed many days of work or school, impacting your education, career, and financial stability. The fatigue and pain can strain relationships as your ability to be intimate or active with partners decreases.

Endometriosis can also lead to infertility if left untreated. As the endometrial tissue builds up, it can distort or block the fallopian tubes and damage reproductive organs. By the time a diagnosis is made, your chances of conceiving naturally may be greatly reduced. This can be devastating for those hoping to start a family.

The late diagnosis also means you've lived with the pain and uncertainty for longer. Not knowing the cause of painful, heavy periods; gastrointestinal issues; or pain during sex for years can take an immense emotional toll. Receiving a diagnosis, although it brings answers, may dredge up feelings of anger at the delay and anxiety over potential treatment options.

The good news is an official diagnosis means you can now work with a doctor to manage symptoms and improve your quality of life. But the lost time can never be recovered, highlighting the need for greater awareness of endometriosis and faster diagnosis and treatment. Through education and advocacy, we can ensure future generations of women do not face the same delays and hardship.

You deserve to live a life free of pain and misunderstanding. Unfortunately, endometriosis often robs women of that basic right for far too long. Don't lose hope - armed with knowledge of the signs and symptoms, you can be your own best advocate. Speak up about your pain and don't stop until you find doctors willing to properly diagnose and treat you. Connect with endometriosis communities to find support and share your story so others don't have to suffer in silence. The lost years may be gone, but there is power in using your voice so that future generations of women no longer have their pain dismissed and lives put on hold. End the delay. End the silence. End endometriosis.

# 21

## THE SILENT KILLER: HOW ENDOMETRIOSIS CLAIMS LIVES

While rarely discussed, endometriosis claims lives in tragic ways. Not only does it drive some to suicide due to intractable pain, but it also spreads in rare cases to vital organs, becoming lethal. affects 1 in 10 women during their reproductive years, yet it often takes years to diagnose and has no cure. The pain it causes can be so agonizing that normal life becomes impossible. Tragically, the social stigma around menstruation and women's health issues has kept endometriosis in the shadows. It's time to bring this silent killer into the light and find ways to detect, treat, and defeat its deadliest forms. Together, we can stop the suffering and save lives.

In rare cases, it may spread beyond the pelvis. This can cause life-threatening complications like intestinal or ureteral blockages. There is also an increased risk of certain cancers, especially ovarian cancer.

Tragically, the severe, chronic pain and life disruption lead some women to take their own lives. The suicide rate for women with endometriosis is 7 times higher than average. Endometriosis needs to be recognized as a serious chronic illness so women can get the treatment, support, and compassion they deserve. Through education and advocacy, we can bring an end to the silent suffering.

Endometrial tissue that escapes the uterus can attach itself to other organs, causing pain, scarring, and damage. The longer endometriosis goes undiagnosed or untreated, the more opportunity it has to spread and worsen.

Endometrial lesions may spread to the ovaries, fallopian tubes, bowels, bladder, and other pelvic structures. This can lead to cysts, adhesions, and scarring that causes organs to stick together. In severe cases, endometriosis can obstruct the bowels or urinary tract.

There is also a risk of endometrial tissue spreading beyond the pelvis to organs like the diaphragm, lungs, and even the brain. While rare, lesions in these locations can cause problems like chest pain, coughing up blood, and seizures.

The damage caused by long-term or untreated endometriosis may require surgery to remove lesions, adhesions, and scar tissue. In some situations, a hysterectomy along with removal of the ovaries and fallopian tubes may be recommended to eliminate the source of the endometrial tissue.

The key is early diagnosis and management of endometriosis. Seeking medical care for pelvic pain and other symptoms can help curb the spread of endometrial tissue before irreparable damage is done. With proper treatment like hormone therapy or excision surgery, most cases of endometriosis can be managed well. However, the more it's allowed to spread, the higher the risks become.

## *The Mental Health Toll: High Rates of Depression and Suicide*

Endometriosis can take a serious mental health toll. Studies show women with endometriosis have higher rates of depression and anxiety, as chronic pain and infertility struggles weigh heavily on both body and mind.

### *High Suicide Risk*

Tragically, endometriosis also increases the risk of suicide. According to research, women with endometriosis are 7 times more likely to commit suicide compared to women without endometriosis.

The severe pain, fertility challenges, lack of treatment options and social isolation are all factors that can contribute to suicidal thoughts in women battling this disease.

## Depression

It's not surprising that endometriosis often leads to depression. The constant pain, medical interventions, financial burden, relationship strain and life disruptions can understandably lead to feelings of sadness, hopelessness and loss of interest in activities. Studies show at least 1 in 3 women with endometriosis also suffer from depression. If you experience symptoms of depression like fatigue, sleep issues, weight changes or thoughts of self-harm, talk to your doctor right away about treatment options such as therapy or medication.

## Anxiety and PTSD

In addition to depression, many women with endometriosis also struggle with anxiety and post-traumatic stress disorder (PTSD). The uncertainty of living with a chronic illness, traumatic medical experiences, infertility fears and lack of control over one's health and body can trigger anxiety and PTSD symptoms like panic attacks, flashbacks and uncontrollable worry. Anti-anxiety medications or counseling may help reduce distressing symptoms.

The psychological impact of endometriosis is very real. Don't hesitate to reach out to loved ones or a mental health professional if you need extra support. And know that you are not alone in what you're going through. There are many resources and communities to help women cope with the mental and emotional challenges of living with this disease.

## *Seeking Support: You Are Not Alone in Your Struggle*

Endometriosis is often referred to as an 'invisible' disease because of the lack of awareness and understanding about its debilitating symptoms. This can make the struggle with endometriosis an incredibly lonely one. However, you are not alone.

Millions of women worldwide suffer from endometriosis. Connecting with others who share your condition can help combat feelings of isolation and provide invaluable support. Here are some ways to build your support network:

- Join an endometriosis support group, either locally or online. Speaking with others who truly understand what you're going through can help alleviate feelings of being alone in your suffering. Facebook has many active endometriosis support groups. Join us at [https://endo-warriors-collective.mn.co/](https://endo-warriors-collective.mn.co/).

- Seek out endometriosis communities on social media. Following accounts dedicated to endometriosis education and awareness is an easy way to stay up-to-date with the latest information about the condition and build camaraderie. Many endometriosis advocates and organizations are active on platforms like Instagram, Twitter and YouTube.

- Tell close friends and family about your condition so they can support you. While endometriosis is still misunderstood by many, educating your close ones about your symptoms and struggles will help them become your allies. Don't suffer in silence.

- Consider counseling or therapy. Speaking with a professional counselor who specializes in chronic health conditions can help you develop coping strategies to better manage the mental and emotional aspects of endometriosis. Therapy can also be useful for overcoming feelings of grief over fertility issues or loss of quality of life.

- Join a support group for infertility or pain management if applicable to your situation. Endometriosis often contributes to issues like infertility, chronic pelvic pain or painful periods. Connecting with others experiencing these challenges can provide support beyond endometriosis alone.

You don't have to go through this alone. Seeking out support from others in the endometriosis community can help give you the strength and solidarity to fight this invisible foe.

## Advocating for Change: Increasing Awareness and Research Funding

Endometriosis is a progressive disease that often goes undiagnosed for years. By the time symptoms become severe enough to seek medical attention, endometrial tissue has typically spread extensively. In some cases, it invades vital organs which can have fatal consequences.

### Organ Failure

Endometriosis causes inflammation and scarring wherever it spreads. When it attacks organs like the lungs, liver, kidneys, and heart, their function becomes impaired. Respiratory failure, liver or kidney disease, and heart attacks have all been linked to endometriosis invading these organs. Treatment options also become more limited and risky once the disease has progressed this far.

### Cancer Risk

Endometriosis also increases the chance of developing certain types of cancer, especially ovarian cancer. According to research, women with endometriosis have up to a 38% higher risk of ovarian cancer compared to the general population. The more severe and long-lasting the endometriosis, the greater the cancer threat becomes.

### *Suicide*

The chronic pain, infertility, hopelessness, and lack of quality of life associated with advanced endometriosis have also been shown to increase the risk of suicide in these patients. Studies report suicide rates up to 7 times higher in women with endometriosis compared to healthy women.

Endometriosis is not just a reproductive health issue but a life-threatening disease. Greater awareness and research funding are desperately needed to develop better diagnostic tools, treatment options, and ultimately a cure. By understanding the true impact endometriosis has on mortality and public health, this hidden epidemic can no longer be ignored. Collectively advocating for political and social change may be the only way to prevent endometriosis from continuing to claim more lives.

The truth is, endometriosis is a silent killer that claims lives in insidious ways. As it spreads throughout your body, it slowly destroys your organs and the very fabric of your being. The chronic pain and suffering caused by this disease drive some to take their own lives to escape the anguish. For others, endometriosis metastasizes to vital organs until they ultimately fail, resulting in premature death.

Endometriosis may start in the uterus, but it does not stay contained there. It is a malignant invader that over time can overtake every part of you. Do not underestimate this disease or think that the pain is normal or will simply go away on its own. Speak up, get the treatment you need, and fight for your health and your life. Endometriosis has already stolen too many futures, do not let it claim yours. There is hope and there are treatments, but early diagnosis and intervention are key. You deserve to live a long, happy, and healthy life free from this silent killer. The time for awareness and action is now.[12]

---

[12] https://www.medicinenet.com/suicidal_thoughts_common_with_endometriosis/news.htm

https://www.ncbi.nlm.nih.gov/pmc/articles/PMC5440042/

https://www.healthline.com/health/can-endometriosis-kill-you

https://www.verywellhealth.com/endometriosis-facts-and-statistics-5324519

https://womenshealth.com.au/endometriosis-suicide/

https://www.ncbi.nlm.nih.gov/pmc/articles/PMC8247611/

https://www.verywellhealth.com/stage-four-endometriosis-7373814

https://www.barnardhealth.us/endometriosis/endometriosis-in-your-brain-rare-but-possible.html

# 22

## ENDOMETRIOSIS AND LOSS OF BODILY AUTONOMY: HOW REPRODUCTIVE RIGHTS AFFECT CHRONIC ILLNESS

As a person with endometriosis, your body often feels like it's no longer your own. The pain, fatigue, and other symptoms associated with this chronic condition can make the simplest acts of living feel like a battle for control. At the same time, society continues to debate and restrict reproductive rights, further limiting your autonomy over your own health and future. For those living with endometriosis, issues like the overturning of Roe v. Wade represent another loss of control over their reproductive systems and medical care.

**The Emotional Toll of Endometriosis**

Living with endometriosis often means grappling with a loss of control over your own body and reproductive rights. The chronic pain and symptoms can be debilitating, disrupting all aspects of your life. On top of the physical difficulties, many endometriosis patients face emotional struggles and mental health issues as a result of the condition.

**The Anxiety and Depression Connection**

Endometriosis is closely linked to anxiety and depression. The constant pain, fatigue, and uncertainty about flare-ups frequently cause worry, stress, and feelings of hopelessness. Studies show endometriosis patients have higher rates of depression and anxiety disorders. The lack of understanding from doctors and loved ones compounds these issues.

## A Sense of Helplessness

The unpredictability of endometriosis leads to a loss of autonomy and helplessness over your own health and body. Not knowing when pain might strike or how long it may last contributes to this loss of control. The limited treatment options also play a role, as many find little relief from available medications and therapies. This helplessness and lack of bodily autonomy has been compared to the loss of freedom experienced with other chronic illnesses.

## Impacts on Relationships and Intimacy

Endometriosis can negatively impact relationships and sex life. Pain during or after intimacy often leads to avoidance of sex, which strains relationships. Fertility issues also contribute, as the desire to get pregnant is hampered by challenges in conceiving. The overall illness and its consequences create obstacles to maintaining a normal sex life and relationships.

While endometriosis manifests physically, its effects are far-reaching. The chronic pain and symptoms lead to a loss of autonomy, helplessness, anxiety, depression, and relationship difficulties. Gaining understanding and support from the medical community and loved ones is vital to improving quality of life and regaining control over your health and body.

## How Restrictive Abortion Laws Affect Those With Endometriosis

For those living with endometriosis, restrictive abortion laws pose a threat to their reproductive rights and bodily autonomy.

### Limited Treatment Options

Those with endometriosis often face limited treatment options, as there is no cure for the condition. Many turn to hormonal contraceptives, like birth control pills, to help manage symptoms and slow the progression of the disease. However, in states with restrictive abortion laws, access to hormonal contraceptives may be limited. This restricts treatment options for those with endometriosis and prevents them from managing a chronic and painful medical condition.

### Impacts on Fertility

Endometriosis can also cause infertility in some cases by blocking the fallopian tubes or ovaries. For those seeking fertility treatments like in vitro fertilization (IVF), restrictive abortion laws may limit access. Some states prohibit fertility treatments that result in unused embryos, while others have attempted to grant "personhood" to embryos, which could outlaw IVF and embryo freezing altogether. This threatens the ability of those with endometriosis to build families.

### Health Complications

In severe cases of endometriosis, a hysterectomy to remove the uterus and ovaries may be recommended as a last resort to relieve symptoms. However, in some states with restrictive abortion laws, access to hysterectomies and other reproductive health procedures may be limited. This could allow endometriosis to continue progressing, causing ongoing health issues like chronic pain, digestive problems, and other complications. I mentioned a while ago that I would explain why Roe Vs. Wade affected me, and this is how.

Restrictive reproductive laws pose a threat to those living with endometriosis by limiting treatment options, impacting fertility, and potentially causing long-term health issues. Protecting reproductive rights is vital for those with chronic illnesses to maintain control over their own health and family planning. Overall, women deserve autonomy over their own bodies and access to the healthcare they need.

## Restricted Reproductive Rights

For endometriosis patients, reproductive rights are complicated by a disease that makes getting pregnant naturally difficult for some. At the same time, conservative policies aim to restrict access to birth control and abortion, limiting options for those with endometriosis to prevent or end an unplanned pregnancy. Some face barriers to hysterectomies or other surgeries that could relieve symptoms when doctors refuse based on a patient's age or childbearing potential.

**Fighting for Recognition and Rights**

The endometriosis community continues to advocate for greater awareness, research funding, and access to healthcare. By speaking out about their experiences with symptoms, diagnosis, and treatment struggles, patients aim to reduce stigma and push for policy changes. Groups lobby lawmakers, organize marches and events, and share educational resources to expand understanding of how endometriosis impacts health, relationships, careers, and daily life.

Together, lack of reproductive rights, chronic pain, and other healthcare obstacles pose serious threats to the autonomy, dignity and quality of life of those living with endometriosis. Through raising their voices, patients are fighting to reclaim power over their own bodies and futures. By listening and working to improve awareness and policy, we can support these efforts to grant endometriosis patients the rights and respect they deserve.

## Resources for Endometriosis Patients in the U.S.

As an endometriosis patient in the U.S., there are several resources available to help you understand your condition and find treatment. Knowing your options can help you gain back some control over your health and quality of life.

### National Endometriosis Foundation

The NEF is a non-profit organization dedicated to promoting endometriosis education, advocacy, support, and research. They offer educational materials on their website to help patients understand diagnosis and treatment options. The NEF also has support groups in many areas of the country, both online and in person. Joining a support group can help combat the isolation that often accompanies chronic illness. You can join our support and educational group at https://endo-warriors-collective.mn.co/.

## Specialist Endometriosis Centers

There are several endometriosis centers located throughout the U.S. that specialize in accurately diagnosing and treating the condition. Centers like the Center for Endometriosis Care, the Endometriosis Institute of America, and the Pearl Women's Center focus specifically on endometriosis and excision surgery. Seeing an endometriosis specialist, especially if you have been struggling to get an accurate diagnosis or effective treatment, may provide the best chance at symptom relief or potential remission.

## Advocacy Organizations

In addition to health resources, there are organizations working to advocate for endometriosis patients and raise awareness of the condition. The Endometriosis Foundation of America works to promote research and education. The Yellow Dress Project brings attention to the condition through public art installations. Working with advocacy groups is a way to make your voice heard and help create change.

## Alternative Treatment Options

For those looking to complement or avoid conventional medical treatment, there are some alternative options to try. Herbal medicine, acupuncture, massage therapy, yoga, and diet changes are some popular alternative treatments for endometriosis. While there is little scientific evidence to support their efficacy, many patients do report symptom relief from these methods. As with any treatment, discuss alternatives with your doctor before proceeding.

The fight against endometriosis can be difficult and exhausting. But by taking advantage of the resources available, you can gain knowledge, find community support, and explore the treatment options that are right for you. Don't lose hope - with self-advocacy, the right care team behind you, and available resources, there are paths to reclaiming your health and autonomy.

## **Coping With Endometriosis in a Changing Political Climate**

Living with endometriosis comes with many challenges, including navigating an unpredictable political climate regarding women's reproductive rights. As states pass laws restricting abortion and birth control access, it can feel disheartening and anxiety-provoking for those with this painful chronic condition. However, there are coping strategies you can employ to feel more in control of your health and future.

### Know Your Rights

Familiarize yourself with laws in your state regarding abortion, birth control, and medical care coverage. While some states have passed restrictive laws, many still protect access to reproductive healthcare services. Talk to your doctor about medical interventions like hormonal contraceptives that can help manage endometriosis symptoms. Stock up on any medications you rely on in case of future restrictions.

### Build Your Support Network

Surround yourself with people who understand what you're going through, whether friends and family or support groups. Online communities for those with endometriosis and chronic illnesses can help combat feelings of isolation. Connecting with others in a similar position helps create solidarity and allows for sharing of advice and resources.

### Engage in Self-Care

Make time for yourself to rest, de-stress and recharge. Try meditation, journaling, art or music therapy, light exercise like yoga, spending time in nature, limiting social media use, etc. Self-care is vital for maintaining your physical and mental health with a condition like endometriosis. Don't feel guilty about putting yourself first.

### Contact Your Representatives

Make your voice heard by writing or calling your political representatives to express how their votes and policies on reproductive rights affect your wellbeing. Share your personal experiences living with endometriosis to put a human face on these issues.

Grassroots advocacy and civic participation can create real change.

While the future of reproductive rights remains uncertain, you can take proactive steps to feel more empowered in coping with endometriosis. Focus on controlling what you can—build your knowledge, support systems and self-care routines. And when you're able, speak up to help shape policies that directly impact your health and access to necessary medical care. Together, we can work to make progress on women's health issues.

## FAQ: Common Questions About Endometriosis and Reproductive Rights

Endometriosis can significantly impact reproductive rights and autonomy over one's own body. Many women face difficult decisions regarding pain management and family planning. It's important to understand how endometriosis and reproductive laws interact.

How does endometriosis affect fertility and pregnancy?

Endometriosis can make it difficult to get pregnant naturally by blocking the fallopian tubes or damaging reproductive organs. Some women require assisted reproductive technology (ART) like in vitro fertilization (IVF) to conceive. Endometriosis may also increase the risk of pregnancy complications. Speak with your doctor about options for fertility treatment and ways to support a healthy pregnancy.

How do abortion laws impact those with endometriosis?

Laws restricting abortion access can limit treatment options for endometriosis-related pain and impact family planning decisions. For example, some women use hormonal contraceptives, like birth control pills, to help reduce endometriosis symptoms in addition to preventing pregnancy. Restrictive laws may limit access to contraceptives. Additionally, in severe cases, women may require surgical procedures that could terminate a pregnancy as a side effect. Strict abortion laws could prevent women from receiving necessary medical care.

What reproductive rights do I have?

Despite facing health challenges, you maintain autonomy over your reproductive health. You have the right to use birth control, pursue fertility treatment, and make decisions regarding pregnancy. However, some laws aim to limit these rights, so stay up to date on legislation in your area. You also have the right to vote for candidates who support women's health and reproductive freedom.

How can I advocate for my rights?

There are many ways to stand up for reproductive rights:

- Contact your political representatives and express your views. Explain how their votes on women's health issues directly impact you.

- Support organizations fighting for reproductive justice like the American Civil Liberties Union (ACLU), Planned Parenthood, and the Endometriosis Foundation of America. Donate or volunteer your time.

- Share your story to raise awareness. Educate others on how endometriosis and reproductive rights are connected. Your experience can help influence opinions and inspire action.

- Vote in all local, state, and federal elections. Make women's health a priority when choosing candidates.

- Join in protests and marches in your area. Come together with others to amplify your collective voice.

- Talk to your doctor about ways they can advocate for patients. Ask them to contact political leaders or sign petitions to support health care access.

By taking action, you can work to expand reproductive rights and ensure all people have control over their own bodies and futures. Don't stay silent—your voice and vote matter.

The pain and uncertainty it causes can make you feel like a prisoner in your own body. Forced to fight for diagnosis and treatment, and faced with limited options to manage symptoms, women with endometriosis often struggle to maintain control over their health and future.

Even after diagnosis, treatment options are imperfect and progress can feel slow. But through advocacy and education, the endometriosis community is working to spread awareness, push for policy changes, and support those newly diagnosed. By speaking up about reproductive rights and demanding better healthcare for chronic illnesses like endometriosis, together we can work to end the loss of bodily autonomy for good. Though the road ahead is long, there is hope.[13]

---

[13] https://www.ncbi.nlm.nih.gov/pmc/articles/PMC9404636/

https://www.linkedin.com/pulse/endometriosis-impact-roe-v-wade-decision-nancy-petersen/

https://nwlc.org/resource/roe-v-wade-and-the-right-to-abortion/

# PART 6

## MEDICATIONS AND TREATMENTS

# 23

# ENDOMETRIOSIS TREATMENT: AN OVERVIEW OF CURRENT OPTIONS TO IMPROVE YOUR LIFE

The good news is we have more treatment choices now than ever before. From pain medication to hormone therapy to minimally invasive surgery, you and your doctor can find the right combination for your needs. While endometriosis can't be cured, it can be managed. Don't lose hope - take charge of your health and explore the possibilities. There are always more options and new research on the horizon. You have the power to ease the pain and get your life back. The road ahead may not be easy, but the destination is worth the journey. Stay strong in your resolve and keep fighting for the care and answers you deserve. There is life beyond the pain, and the treatment is out there to help you find it.

## Hormonal Therapies to Treat Endometriosis

If endometriosis pain is disrupting your life, medication can help provide relief. Several options are available, depending on the severity of your symptoms.

### Over-the-counter pain relievers

For mild to moderate pain, you can try OTC medications like ibuprofen (Advil, Motrin), naproxen (Aleve), or acetaminophen (Tylenol). These reduce inflammation and ease cramps. You may need to take the maximum recommended dose to get relief from endometriosis pain.

### Hormonal birth control

Birth control pills, patches, and rings release hormones that can decrease endometriosis pain. They work by preventing ovulation and reducing inflammation. Many women find their pain is significantly improved with hormonal contraceptives.

### Prescription pain medication

For moderate to severe pain, doctors may prescribe stronger medication like opioids (hydrocodone, oxycodone) or gabapentin (Neurontin). While effective, these also come with risks like dependence or side effects. Only use as directed and under guidance from your physician.

### Hormone therapy

Gonadotropin-releasing hormone (GnRH) agonists shut down the reproductive hormones that stimulate endometriosis growth. They induce a temporary menopause-like state, halting menstruation, and relieving pain. However, side effects like hot flashes and bone loss often limit long term use.

There are many paths to pain relief from endometriosis. Work closely with your doctor to determine the best treatment or combination of therapies based on your unique situation and needs. With the right management plan, you can feel empowered to live comfortably despite this disease.

**Surgical Options for Removing Endometrial Tissue**

Hormonal therapies are commonly used to treat endometriosis and manage pain. These medications work by manipulating your hormone levels to prevent menstruation, reduce inflammation, and slow the growth of endometrial implants. The goal is to create an artificial menopause state or reduce estrogen levels.

## Combined Oral Contraceptives (Birth Control Pills)

Birth control pills contain estrogen and progestin which can help reduce menstrual cramps, pelvic pain, and the growth of endometrial tissue. By preventing ovulation, these pills create an artificial menopause state. Common brands include Yaz, Yasmin, and Ortho Tri-Cyclen.

## Progestins

Progestins, like medroxyprogesterone (Provera) and norethindrone (Aygestin), are synthetic forms of the hormone progesterone. They work by thinning the endometrial lining, reducing inflammation, and slowing the growth of endometrial implants. Progestins are often used for women who can't take estrogen.

## Gonadotropin-Releasing Hormone (GnRH) Agonists

GnRH agonists, such as Lupron and Zoladex, stimulate the release of other hormones that suppress estrogen production by the ovaries. By lowering estrogen levels, they can slow the progression of endometriosis. These drugs often cause menopausal side effects like hot flashes, vaginal dryness, and bone density loss. Add-back therapy with progestins or low-dose estrogen can help reduce these side effects.

### Aromatase Inhibitors

Aromatase inhibitors like Arimidex block the production of estrogen in fat cells and the ovaries. They can be used to treat endometriosis in postmenopausal women or in combination with GnRH agonists. Common side effects include hot flashes, nausea, and joint pain.

These hormone-based treatments may provide relief from symptoms, but endometriosis often returns once treatment is stopped. Surgery is frequently needed to remove endometrial implants and scar tissue for longer-lasting results. A combination of medical and surgical options is typically the most effective approach.

## Complementary Therapies and Lifestyle Changes to Manage Endometriosis

## Surgical Options for Removing Endometrial Tissue

If medication and hormone therapy are not providing enough relief from your endometriosis symptoms, your doctor may recommend surgery. The most common surgeries for endometriosis are:

- Laparoscopy: A minimally invasive procedure where small incisions are made in the abdomen to insert a laparoscope, which is a thin tube with a light and camera. The surgeon can then remove endometrial tissue growths and scar tissue. Laparoscopy has a shorter recovery time than open surgery.

- Hysterectomy: The removal of the uterus. This is usually only recommended in severe cases of endometriosis where other treatments have failed, and pain is chronic. A hysterectomy can provide relief from painful symptoms, but it results in infertility.

- Oophorectomy: The removal of the ovaries. This surgery eliminates the source of estrogen that stimulates endometrial tissue growth. Like a hysterectomy, oophorectomy provides relief from pain but also results in infertility and early menopause.

- Presacral neurectomy: The severing of nerves in the pelvis that transmit pain signals from the uterus and ovaries. This procedure may provide some pain relief but does not treat the underlying endometriosis. Risks include damage to the bowel or bladder.

Endometriosis excision surgery, where endometrial lesions are cut out, has been shown to have better outcomes with lower recurrence rates than procedures that burn or ablate the lesions. An experienced endometriosis specialist can perform meticulous excision of lesions to provide the best chance of relief from symptoms.

Talk to your doctor about which surgical option may be right based on the severity of your condition, your symptoms, age, desire to have children, and other health factors. While surgery does come with risks, for many women it can significantly improve quality of life by reducing pain and restoring fertility. Careful monitoring after surgery is needed to check for recurrence or new growths.

# 24

## THE HIDDEN DANGERS IN TREATING ENDOMETRIOSIS: WHAT YOUR DOCTOR ISN'T TELLING YOU

Chances are, if you're dealing with endometriosis, you've tried more than one medication to relieve the chronic pain and discomfort. You want relief so badly you'll try almost anything the doctor recommends. But what if some of those medications aren't as safe or effective as advertised? New research shows that some common endometriosis treatments can come with hidden dangers and side effects that many doctors don't discuss, leaving you to suffer them unknowingly. As an informed patient, it's important to understand the risks of any treatment before starting it. This chapter will uncover the truth about some of the most popular endometriosis medications, the dangerous side effects they don't warn you about, and safer alternatives you should consider first. You deserve to make the best treatment choices for your body based on the full, unvarnished truth.

## Potential Side Effects and Health Risks of Endometriosis Medications

The medications commonly prescribed for endometriosis may curb symptoms, but they do not provide a cure and often come with unwanted side effects. When taking these drugs long-term, it's important to understand their limitations.

Pain medications like ibuprofen, naproxen, and acetaminophen only provide temporary relief from painful symptoms. They do not slow the progression of the disease or prevent endometriosis from recurring after treatment. After prolonged use, these over-the-counter drugs can cause stomach issues or kidney/liver damage.

Hormonal birth control, including the pill, patch, ring, and hormonal IUD aim to prevent menstruation which can temporarily suppress endometriosis. However, once you stop taking them, symptoms often return within months. These contraceptives also frequently cause unwanted side effects like mood changes, weight gain, acne, and loss of libido.

Lupron Depot, a GnRH agonist, induces a temporary menopause to relieve endometriosis symptoms. However, "menopause" comes with hot flashes, bone loss, and other issues. Add-back therapy with hormones may reduce side effects but does not eliminate them. Like other medications, Lupron does not provide a permanent solution. Endometriosis will likely flare up again once treatment stops.

Surgery, especially excision of endometriosis lesions, is currently considered the gold standard for treating endometriosis and improving quality of life. However, even with the most skilled surgeon, endometriosis can recur in up to 50% of women within 5-10 years following surgery. Repeat surgeries also increase risks.

The harsh reality is endometriosis is a chronic illness with no straightforward remedy. A multidisciplinary approach combining medication, surgery, lifestyle changes, and complementary therapies provides the best odds of managing symptoms long-term. But there is still no guarantee of being pain-free or preventing recurrence. Ongoing monitoring and a willingness to try different options is key. The best we can hope for, at this point in time, is effectively managing the condition to maximize quality of life.

**Exploring Alternative and Complementary Therapies for Endometriosis Management**

The medications commonly prescribed for endometriosis may provide relief from symptoms, but they also come with risks and side affects you should be aware of.

## Hormonal birth control

Birth control pills, patches and rings are often used to suppress menstruation and decrease pain. However, they may cause nausea, headaches, weight gain, and mood changes. Long term use or high estrogen doses can increase the risk of blood clots, high blood pressure, and certain types of cancer.

## GnRH agonists

These injectable drugs prevent ovulation and menstruation but often cause menopause-like side effects such as hot flashes, vaginal dryness, and bone loss. They should not be used long term due to these risks.

## Nexplanon

The progesterone implant Nexplanon can reduce pain but frequently leads to irregular or non-stop bleeding that may require medication to control. It can also cause acne, headaches, and weight gain in some women.

## Lupron

Lupron injections block estrogen production to induce a temporary menopause state. While it may decrease endometriosis pain, it commonly causes severe menopause symptoms that can significantly impact quality of life. It also poses risks like bone loss and memory issues with long term use.

## Surgery

Laparoscopic surgery to remove endometriosis lesions and scar tissue can provide longer-lasting relief than medications alone. However, surgery does come with risks like infection, blood loss, damage to other organs. Repeat surgeries may be needed for recurrence, and endometriosis can still return even after surgery.

While medications and surgery aim to manage symptoms and slow disease progression, there is currently no cure for endometriosis. The options available often require finding the treatment or combination of treatments with side affects you can live with, while maximizing your quality of life. Discussing the pros, cons and alternatives with your doctor can help determine the best path forward based on your priorities and health needs.

# 25

## ENDING THE SILENCE: GIVING WOMEN WITH ENDOMETRIOSIS A VOICE

The lack of awareness about endometriosis among physicians and the general public, insufficient funding for research, and the normalization of period pain as something women just have to endure all contribute to this long, frustrating journey for answers and relief that too many women find themselves on. Ending the silence around endometriosis and improving education and resources are urgently needed to provide better support for those affected.

## Emerging Research on New Treatment Options

Getting an endometriosis diagnosis and effective treatment can be frustratingly difficult. There are several barriers' women face along the way:

### Lack of Awareness

Endometriosis is not openly discussed, so many women and even doctors do not fully understand the condition or recognize the symptoms. The average woman sees 5 doctors over 9 years before being diagnosed.

### Menstrual Pain Normalized

Severe pain with menstruation is often dismissed as "just cramps" or normal female troubles. But if pain is debilitating, long-lasting, or does not improve with over-the-counter medication, it could indicate endometriosis.

## Invisibility of the Disease

Since endometriosis cannot be seen with the naked eye, some doctors may wrongly assume a woman's pain is psychological or make her feel like she's exaggerating. A diagnosis requires laparoscopic surgery to view the reproductive organs.

## Treatment Limitations

Treatment options are limited and often come with undesirable side effects like menopausal symptoms. Hormone therapy and surgery may only provide temporary relief. More research is urgently needed to find better solutions for managing this chronic disease.

## Cost and Access

Diagnosis and treatment can be expensive and time-consuming, especially if multiple doctors are seen. Many women struggle to get diagnosis and care due to lack of insurance, financial hardship, or simply not having options in their area.

Endometriosis needs to be brought out of the shadows. With increased awareness, understanding and advocacy, women can receive faster diagnosis and better access to comprehensive treatment. Their pain can be validated and managed so they can live full, productive lives.

**Improving Access to Care Through Policy Changes**

**Emerging Research on New Treatment Options**

As awareness of endometriosis grows, so does funding for research into new treatment options. Here are some of the promising areas currently being investigated:

### Hormonal Treatments

- New hormonal contraceptives are in development to better control menstruation and reduce inflammation without the side effects of current birth control pills.

- Gonadotropin-releasing hormone (GnRH) antagonists are also being studied to block estrogen production in a more targeted way.

## Immunotherapy

- Immunomodulators that can alter the immune system's response are showing potential for reducing inflammation and pain.

- Clinical trials are underway for medications like leuprolide that may inhibit the production of inflammatory prostaglandins.

## Surgical Options

- Improvements in minimally invasive surgery techniques like laparoscopy are making surgery safer, with shorter recovery times.

- New methods for destroying endometrial lesions with heat, cold or laser are also in development to provide an alternative to excision surgery.

**Lifestyle Therapies**

- Acupuncture, massage therapy, yoga and diet changes may provide non-medical ways to relieve symptoms.

- Preliminary research shows promise for anti-inflammatory diets, pelvic floor therapy, and Traditional Chinese Medicine.

More research is still desperately needed, but there are hopeful signs on the horizon. By advocating for continued funding and participating in clinical trials, you can help accelerate progress toward more effective and accessible treatment options. Together, we can work to ensure that women with endometriosis get the care and respect they deserve.

**Stories From Women Living with Endometriosis**

**Improving Access to Care Through Policy Changes**

While endometriosis affects an estimated 1 in 10 women, many struggle to get diagnosed and find effective treatment. Policy changes could help make care more accessible.

To start, educating doctors and healthcare providers about endometriosis is key. Requiring endometriosis education and training for all OB/GYNs and family physicians would ensure they know how to properly diagnose and treat the condition. Early diagnosis and intervention are critical, as endometriosis can worsen over time without treatment.

Increasing research funding for endometriosis is also needed. There are still too many unknowns about the causes and progression of the disease. Additional funding would support research for more targeted treatment options with fewer side effects. Non-invasive diagnostic tools are also needed to reduce reliance on surgery for diagnosis.

Improving insurance coverage for endometriosis care would help many women access necessary treatment. Endometriosis treatments like excision surgery, hormone therapy, pain management, and fertility treatments should be covered as essential health benefits. Out-of-pocket costs keep many women from getting the care they need.

Advocating for policy changes with lawmakers and healthcare organizations is key. Grassroots campaigns and nonprofit groups are working to raise awareness of issues around endometriosis care and put pressure on policymakers. Individual women can also contact their political representatives to share their experiences and call for improved access to diagnosis and treatment.

Collective action can drive real change. While endometriosis may still be misunderstood, women deserve access to high-quality care. Policy changes, education, research, and advocacy are all needed to make that access a reality. No woman should suffer in silence or go without the care she needs. Together, we can work to end the silence on endometriosis.

# PART 7

FUNDING AND RESEARCH

# 26

## FIGHTING AN INVISIBLE ENEMY: NAVIGATING THE FUNDING MAZE FOR ENDOMETRIOSIS RESEARCH

As a woman struggling with endometriosis, you know firsthand how debilitating and painful this condition can be. Despite affecting over 176 million women worldwide, endometriosis remains an underfunded, often misunderstood disease. For decades, research into its causes and potential treatments has moved at a glacial pace. But recently, new funding initiatives are helping accelerate progress. Learn about the major players driving endometriosis research today and how their efforts are unlocking new insights into this complex disorder. Together, by supporting organizations championing endometriosis research and advocacy, we can help build momentum and find answers for millions of women living with this disease. The road ahead is long, but at last we have reasons to hope.

The physical, emotional, and financial toll of endometriosis can be overwhelming. Patients report spending over $10,000 per year in out-of-pocket medical costs on average. They make lifestyle changes and sacrifice activities they enjoy in order to manage pain. Too often, endometriosis leads to feelings of isolation, loss of self-worth and strained relationships.

Through advocacy and education, the endometriosis community is working to raise awareness of the life-altering effects of this disease and the urgent need for non-invasive diagnosis, more treatment options, and ultimately, a cure. Patients deserve nothing less.

## Types of Organizations Supporting Endometriosis Research

Endometriosis affects an estimated 1 in 10 women during their reproductive years, yet research funding for this debilitating disease remains disproportionately low. According to recent analyses, endometriosis receives less than half the funding of other similarly prevalent diseases.

### Current Funding Levels

Endometriosis research is primarily funded through public agencies like the National Institutes of Health (NIH) in the US, as well as private organizations such as the Endometriosis Foundation of America (EFA) and Endometriosis Research Center (ERC). However, combined funding from these sources amounts to only around $11 million per year - a tiny fraction of the funding for diseases with similar prevalence.

For women struggling with endometriosis, the lack of research funding is frustrating and disheartening. More funding is desperately needed to better understand the causes and mechanisms of this enigmatic disease, improve diagnosis, and develop more effective treatments. Increased funding could accelerate research in key areas like:

- The search for non-invasive diagnostic biomarkers to eliminate the need for surgery

- Clinical trials of emerging medical therapies to expand treatment options

- Basic research on the genetic and hormonal factors underlying endometriosis

- Improved patient education and support programs

While advocacy organizations work to raise awareness of endometriosis and lobby for increased research funding, individuals can also make a difference by donating to and volunteering with organizations that fund endometriosis research. Together, we can unlock answers and open up new avenues of hope for the millions of women living with this invisible illness.

## Emerging Areas of Focus in Endometriosis Research

There are several types of organizations that provide funding for endometriosis research.

## Non-Profits

Endometriosis foundations and charities, such as the Endometriosis Foundation of America (EFA) and the World Endometriosis Society (WES), provide grants and fellowships for endometriosis research. The EFA has funded over $10 million in research since its inception. These non-profits rely on donations and fundraising to support research.

## Government Agencies

Government organizations like the National Institutes of Health (NIH) and the Patient-Centered Outcomes Research Institute (PCORI) offer grants for endometriosis research in the U.S. The NIH is the largest public funder of endometriosis research, awarding over $114 million in grants over the past 20 years. PCORI focuses on comparative clinical effectiveness research and patient-centered outcomes research.

## Academic Institutions

Many universities have endometriosis research programs that are funded through government grants as well as private donations. For example, the University of California San Francisco has an endometriosis research program focusing on genetics, immunology, and novel treatments. Academic institutions are instrumental in training the next generation of endometriosis researchers and physicians.

## Biotech and Pharmaceutical Companies

Biotechnology and pharmaceutical companies that develop new treatments for endometriosis help fund research through investments in early-stage research, clinical trials, and partnerships with non-profits and academic institutions. For example, AbbVie, which makes Orilissa, partners with RESOLVE: The National Infertility Association to fund research grants. Increased private sector investment in endometriosis research is still needed to drive innovation.

While funding for endometriosis research has grown over the years, endometriosis is still an underfunded condition relative to its prevalence and impact. Continued support from a variety of sources is critical to improving diagnosis, developing better treatments, and ultimately finding a cure.

## Emerging Areas of Focus in Endometriosis Research

As researchers work to unlock the mysteries of endometriosis, several promising areas of focus are emerging.

### Hormonal Influences

Endometriosis is an estrogen-dependent disease, meaning estrogen stimulates the growth of endometrial tissue outside the uterus. Researchers are exploring ways to block estrogen's effects on endometriotic lesions and slow their progression. Promising options include selective estrogen receptor modulators (SERMs) and aromatase inhibitors.

### Inflammation

Endometriosis is associated with inflammation in the pelvis. Researchers are studying anti-inflammatory medications and natural compounds to reduce inflammation in endometriosis-affected tissues. Preliminary research shows benefits from omega-3 fatty acids, turmeric or curcumin supplements, and non-steroidal anti-inflammatory drugs (NSAIDs) like ibuprofen.

## Immune System Dysfunction

The immune system plays a role in the development and spread of endometriosis. Researchers are exploring ways to regulate the immune system and correct any dysfunction that may contribute to disease progression. Options include immune-regulating medications, probiotics, and prebiotics to balance gut bacteria, and lifestyle changes like stress reduction techniques.

## Genetics

Family history is a significant risk factor for endometriosis, suggesting genetics are involved. By identifying specific genes linked to endometriosis risk, researchers can better understand the mechanisms driving the disease and develop targeted treatments. Recent genome-wide association studies have identified multiple genetic variants associated with endometriosis risk.

Continued research funding and advocacy are critical to accelerating progress in these areas. With increased understanding of the complex interplay between hormones, inflammation, immunity, genetics, and environment in endometriosis, we move closer to finding life-changing solutions for those affected.

# 27

# ENDOMETRIOSIS FUNDING: WHY THE NEGLECT?

## Comparing Funding for Endometriosis to Other Diseases

Endometriosis affects an estimated 1 in 10 women, yet research and funding lag far behind other conditions. Compared to illnesses like breast cancer, endometriosis receives a tiny fraction of research funding despite the significant costs in healthcare and lost work productivity.

Endometriosis has a debilitating impact on women and the economy. The average patient takes 9.2 years to be properly diagnosed and incurs annual healthcare costs over $10,000. Lost work hours cost $12 billion per year in the U.S. alone. Yet in 2017, endometriosis garnered only $7 million in NIH research funding while breast cancer received $698 million.

The lack of research means limited treatment options and understanding of the condition. The average patient tries 4 doctors and 5 treatments before finding relief. Available treatments often come with severe side effects like menopause, and recurrence rates are high.

More funding and research are urgently needed. Researchers could gain insights into the causes and progression, leading to earlier diagnosis and more effective treatments with fewer side effects. With increased awareness and education, doctors may be better equipped to identify and manage symptoms.

Women with endometriosis deserve the same medical support and quality of life as those with better-understood conditions. It's time to correct the neglect and make endometriosis a higher priority in research funding and public health education. Together, we can bring this invisible illness into the light.

**Reasons for the Funding Disparity**

Comparing the funding for endometriosis to other medical conditions reveals a startling discrepancy. Endometriosis affects roughly the same number of women as diabetes, yet diabetes receives over 60 times more research funding from the National Institutes of Health (NIH).

Endometriosis causes tissue similar to the lining of the uterus to grow outside of the uterus, leading to severe pain, infertility, and other symptoms that disrupt quality of life. The pain from endometriosis is frequently compared to cancer pain. Despite the significant physical and emotional toll, endometriosis receives only $11 million per year in NIH funding.

- Diabetes, which impacts a comparable number of people in the U.S., receives $674 million annually from NIH for research.

- Alzheimer's disease impacts 5.8 million Americans and receives $2.4 billion in NIH funding.

- Lung cancer, with 228,000 new cases each year, receives $352 million.

The lack of funding for endometriosis is an example of the inequality that still exists in women's health research. Diseases primarily impacting women have long been underfunded and understudied. Endometriosis advocates have campaigned for years to close this gap, arguing it should be a higher priority given its significant health burden and the potential benefits of improved treatments. Increased research could help develop less invasive diagnostic tools, more effective treatments with fewer side effects, and possibly even a cure.

While all diseases deserve research funding, the enormous disparity for endometriosis is unacceptable and limits progress that could relieve suffering for millions of women. Closing this gap should be a top priority to improve women's health. Overall, endometriosis funding needs a massive boost to provide this generation and the next with better options and quality of life.

Endometriosis is a painful disorder in which tissue similar to the lining of the uterus grows outside of the uterus. Despite affecting an estimated 1 in 10 women during their reproductive years, endometriosis receives a disproportionately small amount of research funding. Here are a few reasons why this funding disparity exists:

Endometriosis remains poorly understood and under-diagnosed. Many women suffer for years before receiving an accurate diagnosis and treatment. This lack of awareness and understanding has contributed to endometriosis being viewed as a "niche" condition rather than a priority for research investment.

Diseases that primarily affect women often face discrimination in the medical community and research field. Endometriosis has long been dismissed as "just painful periods" and not taken seriously as a debilitating disorder warranting research attention.

Endometriosis research struggles to receive funding through traditional means like government grants. The review committees that determine funding priorities frequently lack expertise in women's reproductive health issues. Researchers also face challenges convincing funding organizations that endometriosis research could have broad applications and benefits.

The endometriosis community has lacked a strong, unified advocacy voice to raise awareness and lobby for increased research funds the way other health conditions have done. Building up advocacy and lobbying efforts is critical to overcoming the systemic barriers facing endometriosis research.

While the funding situation remains dire, continued advocacy and education offer hope for change. By raising our voices together, we can push endometriosis to the forefront and make reproductive health issues a priority. Increased funds would allow for improved diagnosis, treatment, and ultimately, a cure.

# 28

## THE HIGH PRICE OF ENDOMETRIOSIS: HOW LACK OF RESEARCH FUNDING LIMITS TREATMENT OPTIONS

The chronic pain and uncertainty take an enormous psychological and emotional toll. Relationships, careers, and daily activities are impacted. Yet endometriosis receives only a fraction of the research funding of other chronic illnesses, estimated at less than 2% of funding for conditions of similar prevalence.

Without more funding, improved diagnostic tools, treatment options, and ultimately a cure will remain elusive. Despite the enormous costs to individuals and society, endometriosis continues to be under-researched and misunderstood. For women battling this invisible illness, more research funding means hope - the hope of being able to reclaim their lives, start a family, and live without pain. The hope of a future free from endometriosis.

For decades, endometriosis research has been crippled by lack of funding. The National Institutes of Health (NIH) spends only $11 million annually on endometriosis research - a tiny fraction of funding for other diseases that affect similar numbers of women. Without research, diagnosis takes an average of 7-12 years. Treatment options are limited to hormonal birth control and surgery, which often only provide temporary relief from painful symptoms.

For endometriosis sufferers, this means a lower quality of life and fewer opportunities. The continuous pain and flare-ups disrupt work, education, relationships, and daily activities. Many women struggle to maintain employment due to excessive sick days and medical appointments. The high cost of out-of-pocket medical expenses also places a huge financial burden on those affected.

Increased funding for research is desperately needed to improve diagnosis, find better treatment options, and ultimately, uncover a cure. Researchers have promising leads but lack the funding to thoroughly explore them. With more funding, research could accelerate understanding and developing of new nonsurgical treatments, less invasive surgeries, and ways to prevent recurrence.

Endometriosis may be a silent disease, but the suffering is loud and clear. It's time to speak up and make endometriosis research funding a priority. Women deserve so much more than to be told pain is normal or in their heads. They deserve real answers and real solutions. Increased research funding can make that a reality.

The lack of funding for endometriosis research has severely limited treatment options for patients. With meager research budgets, scientists struggle to make meaningful progress in understanding the mechanisms driving this complex disease.

Currently, there are few good treatment options for endometriosis beyond hormonal contraceptives, pain medication, and invasive surgery. These options only provide temporary relief and do nothing to slow disease progression. Because the disease is so poorly understood, developing new targeted treatments has been nearly impossible.

Research progress moves at a glacial pace due to lack of funding. It can take many years to gather enough data to gain insights or test new hypotheses. Clinical trials for potential new treatments often stall or are cancelled due to lack of funding. Women continue to suffer through years of pain, infertility, and poor quality of life while waiting for answers.

With more funding, researchers could make use of advanced technologies like genomic sequencing, biobanking, and precision medicine to gain insights into the genetics of endometriosis. They could identify new drug targets and biomarkers to enable earlier diagnosis. Additional funding would allow more researchers to devote their time and expertise to studying this disease, accelerating progress.

While endometriosis is estimated to affect 1 in 10 women, research funding levels do not match the scale of this issue. Patients, advocacy groups, and researchers continue to appeal for more public and private funding to drive progress in understanding and treating this debilitating disease. With more funding, the future could hold targeted treatments, improved surgery, biomarkers for early diagnosis, and even prevention. But without it, women will continue to suffer in silence, waiting for the answers that more research could provide.

# PART 8

ADVOCACY AND ACTION

# 29

## ADVOCACY OUTREACH: A CALL TO ACTION FOR ENDOMETRIOSIS AWARENESS

Endometriosis can have a significant impact on patients' quality of life. The chronic pain and discomfort caused by this condition often leads to:

- Difficulty with daily activities like exercising, socializing, and working. The pain from endometriosis can be debilitating, making even simple tasks challenging.

- Sleep problems and fatigue. The constant pain disrupts sleep, and the lack of rest worsens symptoms like low energy, impaired concentration, and mood changes.

- Emotional stress and mental health issues. Living with endometriosis may increase the risk of anxiety, depression, and other psychological conditions due to the physical distress and life disruptions.

- Relationship difficulties. Endometriosis can strain intimate relationships by causing pain during sex, reduced libido, and fertility problems. Partners may have trouble understanding what patients are going through.

- Career and education impacts. Missing work or school because of endometriosis symptoms can threaten job security, career progression, and academic success. Some women have had to make major life changes to accommodate their condition.

The severity of endometriosis and the specific symptoms experienced by each patient will determine how significantly their life is affected. But due to the chronic and often invisible nature of this disease, raising awareness about the potential impacts can help foster understanding and support. Patients deserve compassion and accommodation, so they have the best chance to thrive despite their diagnosis. Together, we can make a difference through education and advocacy.

There are several advocacy organizations working to raise awareness of endometriosis and support those affected. These groups aim to educate the public and medical community about this painful disorder in order to improve diagnosis, treatment, and quality of life.

### Endometriosis Foundation of America

The EFA promotes research, education, and advocacy. They work with congressional representatives to gain support for legislation like the Endometriosis Research Center of Excellence Act. The EFA also provides education for healthcare providers and funds research grants.

## World Endometriosis Society

The WES is an international organization that brings together healthcare professionals and researchers focused on endometriosis. They host conferences, publish reports, and work to establish standards of care. The WES also provides training and education for physicians to improve diagnosis and treatment.

## Endometriosis Network Canada

ENC provides support and education for those with endometriosis in Canada. They work to raise public awareness, advocate for improved healthcare policies, and fund research. ENC has also established support groups and an online community for those living with endometriosis.

## EndoFound

EndoFound focuses on advocacy and raising awareness about endometriosis. They work with legislators to pass resolutions officially recognizing March as Endometriosis Awareness Month. EndoFound also promotes education in schools and provides resources for talking to friends and family about the disease. They aim to reduce stigma and empower those with endometriosis to speak up about their condition.

These organizations, along with local support groups, are making a difference through advocacy and action. By raising awareness, promoting education, and calling for policy changes, they are working to build a better future for everyone affected by endometriosis. There are many ways to get involved, from donating to volunteering your time. Together, we can make a difference.

## Spreading Awareness Through social media and Community Outreach

There are many ways you can get involved to raise awareness and advocate for the endometriosis community. Every action makes a difference in driving change.

### Contact your political representatives.

Let your local, state, and federal government officials know that endometriosis research and treatment needs to be a priority. Call or write to express your support for legislation that funds endometriosis research and treatment, as well as affordable care.

### Participate in awareness campaigns

Get involved in national endometriosis campaigns like EndoMarch to raise public awareness. You can organize or join community walks, share information on social media, write blog posts or letters to the editor for local media, or volunteer your time.

### Educate others

One of the biggest challenges of endometriosis is lack of understanding. Educate family, friends, healthcare providers, and others in your community about the signs and symptoms of endometriosis and the latest treatment options. Share resources from reputable endometriosis organizations.

### Join a local support group

Find an endometriosis support group in your area or start your own. Support groups are a great way to connect with others who share your experience, learn coping strategies, and organize awareness efforts together. Many organizations offer resources to help start a support group.

### Participate in research studies

Volunteering for clinical trials, surveys and other research studies is one of the best ways to advance endometriosis research and new treatment options. Look for opportunities at local universities, hospitals, and research institutions in your area. You can also sign up on websites like EndoFound.org.

Every action makes a difference in creating change. By raising your voice and participating in advocacy and awareness, you can help improve quality of life for all those affected by endometriosis. Together, we can drive progress.

# 30

# A SYMPHONY OF VOICES: PATIENTS, PROVIDERS AND POLICYMAKERS DRIVING HEALTHCARE REFORM

A transformation is underway in healthcare, fueled by the voices of those directly impacted. Patients are sharing their experiences to highlight what's working, what's not, and what needs to change. Healthcare providers are advocating for reforms allowing them to provide the best care possible. And forward-thinking policymakers are listening, crafting innovative solutions to make the system more equitable and effective.

Progress is being made, but more voices are still needed. Yours, mine, all of ours. Together, our chorus for change is building into a symphony with the power to shape a healthcare system we can all believe in. One that treats patients as partners, gives providers the freedom to do their best work, and takes policy in a direction that benefits us all. The future of healthcare reform will be defined by the voices of patients, providers, and policymakers - together, advocating as one.

Patients are uniquely positioned to advocate for change in the healthcare system. By sharing their experiences, stories, and perspectives, patients can raise awareness of important issues and put pressure on providers and policymakers to drive reform.

As patients navigate the healthcare system, they gain firsthand knowledge about what's working and what needs improvement. Patients can use their voices to call out inefficiencies, lack of coordination, or subpar care. For example, a patient may speak up about excessive wait times, confusing billing practices, or lack of empathy from staff.

Patients should share experiences on social media or write letters to healthcare organizations, political representatives, and media outlets. Patients can also join local advocacy groups to make their voices louder and lobby for new laws and policies.

Personal stories and experiences are compelling ways to highlight challenges in the system and rally support for change. By sharing a story about a medical error, lack of access to treatment, or financial hardship due to medical bills, patients can elicit emotion and prompt action. Patients should share stories on platforms like health advocacy websites, social media, blogs, podcasts, and with local media.

While speaking up as an individual is impactful, patients can achieve more by banding together. Patient advocacy organizations provide opportunities to share stories, exchange ideas, learn best practices, and take collective action. Working together, the patient community has the power to drive meaningful and lasting healthcare reform.

As healthcare providers, you have a wealth of knowledge and experience that can drive meaningful change. By advocating for your patients and profession, you can influence policymakers and healthcare organizations to make decisions that truly support patient care.

Through research and data analysis, providers identify care gaps and solutions. For example, a survey may show patients struggle accessing mental healthcare in your area. Armed with these insights, providers can propose policy changes to improve access, whether increasing funding for community health centers or incentivizing psychiatrists to work in underserved regions.

Providers may be called upon to testify before local, state, or federal government committees. Sharing your expertise and stories from the frontlines of care can help policymakers understand the real-world impacts of their decisions. Your voice lends credibility and urgency, motivating them to pursue patient-centered reforms.

Doctors and nurses can also lead by example through community outreach and education. Speaking at schools, writing blog posts or newspaper editorials, and participating in public forums are ways to raise awareness of health issues, combat misinformation, and encourage healthy behaviors.

While policy change often happens gradually, each action providers take - conducting research, advocating for patients, building community trust - moves us closer to a healthcare system centered on human needs and values. By adding your voice, experience, and passion as advocates, you can be instrumental in achieving greater access, equity, and quality of care for all.

Policymakers play an instrumental role in healthcare reform by introducing and advocating for legislation aimed at improving the system. As elected officials, they are in a position to propose and push for laws that increase access, lower costs, and value patients' needs.

In recent years, policymakers have championed several bills focused on patient-centered reform. The Affordable Care Act, passed in 2010, expanded health insurance to millions of Americans by prohibiting denial of coverage due to pre-existing conditions, allowing young adults to stay on their parents' plans until age 26, and providing subsidies for low-income individuals.

Other proposed legislation like the Patient Protection Act aims to curb surprise billing, cap out-of-pocket costs for prescription drugs, and require insurance companies to provide upfront price estimates. The bill's sponsors argue it will shield patients from unanticipated high costs and make the healthcare system more transparent.

Policymakers are also working to address broader issues around cost and inequality. Some support a "Medicare for All" system which would provide universal healthcare funded by taxpayers. Others propose a public option to compete with private plans or policies targeting specific costs like drug prices.

Reform-minded policymakers recognize that substantial change is still needed to achieve a healthcare system that puts patients first and values health over profits. By giving voice to the challenges Americans face in accessing and affording care, elected officials have the power to craft legislative solutions that balance the interests of all stakeholders. While progress can be slow, continued advocacy and compromise from policymakers are crucial to driving system-wide improvements that benefit both

When patients, healthcare providers, and policymakers come together around a shared goal, their collective voices are amplified, and real change can happen. By building coalitions and alliances, these key stakeholders can educate lawmakers and the public, put pressure on

Patients and physicians who have firsthand experience with health issues can share their stories with legislators and government officials. Their testimonies about living with a condition or lacking critical resources often resonate more than statistics alone. Healthcare providers also have a duty to advocate for evidence-based policymaking and speak out against harmful legislation. Educating elected officials and policymakers is key to crafting laws and regulations that actually meet people's needs.

While patients, physicians, hospitals, and health systems each have their own priorities, finding common ground and a shared vision for change can make their message much more powerful. Collaborating on advocacy campaigns, drafting joint position statements, and signing on to each other's calls for action are effective ways to show solidarity and build momentum behind key issues. Speaking with one voice makes it difficult for policymakers and leaders to ignore their demands or dismiss their concerns.

Once stakeholders have a unified message, they can take collective action to put pressure on healthcare systems, government agencies, and elected officials. Things like petitions, protests, sit-ins, strikes, and boycotts have historically been useful tactics for raising awareness of critical problems, conveying the urgency of the situation, and forcing the hand of decision makers. While these methods can be controversial, they are often a last resort when other attempts at negotiation and compromise have failed.

By working together, patients, healthcare providers, and policymakers can drive real reforms and make the healthcare system better serve all those who rely on it. Through education, developing a shared vision, and applying pressure when needed, their collective voice becomes difficult to ignore.

# 31

## WINNING THE ENDOMETRIOSIS BATTLE: A COMPREHENSIVE STRATEGY FOR ADVANCEMENT

By raising awareness of endometriosis, we can help women identify its signs earlier and seek proper treatment and support. Public awareness campaigns should focus on common symptoms like painful periods, painful intercourse, chronic pelvic pain, and infertility.

Promoting open discussions about menstruation and women's health issues will help end the stigma surrounding endometriosis. We need to share info about endometriosis on social media, create informative videos and podcasts, and pitch stories to media outlets.

### Improving Healthcare Education

Doctors and nurses should receive better education on properly diagnosing and treating endometriosis. Many women suffer for years before receiving an accurate diagnosis and treatment. We must advocate for improved endometriosis education at medical schools and provide continuing education for practicing physicians.

With increased public awareness and enhanced healthcare education, more women can get diagnosed sooner and receive the necessary care and treatment to manage symptoms and slow disease progression.

Together, we can win the fight against this "silent epidemic".

## Improving Access to Specialized Care and Multi-Disciplinary Teams

To increase funding and spur more rapid advancement in endometriosis research and treatment, we must advocate to politicians, healthcare organizations, and research institutes. Our voices have power, and together we can drive real change.

Contact your political representatives and ask them to support bills that provide funding for endometriosis research and education. Explain how this chronic disease impacts over 176 million women worldwide - likely someone in their life as well. Urge them to make this a priority issue.

Reach out to healthcare groups and encourage them to provide education on endometriosis for physicians, nurses, and staff. Early diagnosis and proper treatment can make a world of difference for sufferers. Ask that they also support related legislation and donate to research.

Write letters to research hospitals and institutes. Describe your endometriosis journey and the lack of knowledge and options available. Appeal to them to make endometriosis a primary research focus, as too little is understood about its causes and the most effective treatments. More clinical studies are desperately needed.

Share your story on social media using the hashtag #EndoAdvocacy to raise public awareness. Tag politicians, healthcare organizations and research institutes to increase visibility and spur action. United, our voices can influence real change.

By taking these steps to advocate for more funding, research, education, and resources focused on endometriosis, we move closer to better treatment options and ultimately a cure. Staying silent will not bring solutions - we must speak up and demand a better future for the millions affected by this debilitating disease. Together, we can win this battle.

## Developing New and Better Medications and Treatments

Improving access to specialized endometriosis care and multi-disciplinary medical teams is crucial for advancement. Right now, an estimated 10% of women suffer from endometriosis, but many go undiagnosed for up to 10 years due to lack of awareness and available expertise.

To increase access to specialized endometriosis care, we need more gynecologists and surgeons trained in the latest diagnosis and treatment techniques. Promoting awareness of fellowship programs and encouraging doctors to specialize in endometriosis and pelvic pain will help build this workforce.

Regional endometriosis centers of excellence with multi-disciplinary teams including gynecologists, surgeons, pain specialists, nutritionists and physical therapists are ideal for providing comprehensive care. These centers can also conduct research and clinical trials on new treatments. Nonprofits and private donors should support the launch and ongoing funding of more endometriosis centers across the country.

Telemedicine and virtual consults with endometriosis specialists provide another avenue for access when in-person care isn't available. Remote monitoring options let women connect regularly with their doctor via online video or messaging. Specialists can review symptoms, test results, and make adjustments to treatment plans when needed. Offering telemedicine services at lower or no-cost for endometriosis patients provides access for those unable to travel or pay out-of-pocket expenses.

Endometriosis education and support programs are crucial for helping women navigate their diagnosis and available treatment options. Patient advocacy organizations can develop programs to spread awareness, equip women with questions to ask their doctors, and connect them with local resources. Providing education and support will empower women to advocate for the best care possible.

Together, increasing specialized practitioners, establishing regional centers of excellence, utilizing telemedicine, and providing education and support programs will significantly improve access to high-quality endometriosis care. No woman should have to suffer in silence or travel far from home to find the treatment she deserves. With a coordinated strategy, we can make vital endometriosis care available to all who need it.

## Providing Holistic Support for Those Suffering from Endometriosis

Developing new and improved treatments for endometriosis is critical to reducing suffering and helping those affected live full lives. Several promising areas of research could lead to better medications and therapies.

### Hormonal Treatments

Hormone therapy aims to interrupt the menstrual cycle and reduce estrogen levels that fuel the growth of endometrial tissue outside the uterus. Existing hormonal options like birth control pills, patches and intrauterine devices can help manage symptoms for some, but often come with undesirable side effects. Researchers are working on more targeted hormone treatments with fewer side effects, such as selective progesterone receptor modulators (SPRMs). These drugs block the action of progesterone only in the endometrium and endometriotic lesions.

## Immunotherapy

The immune system plays a role in the development and spread of endometriosis. Immunotherapy uses medications to modify or harness the immune system to treat disease. For endometriosis, researchers are investigating ways to block the formation of new blood vessels that feed endometrial tissue growth (anti-angiogenesis therapy), target inflammation and immune responses that promote disease (anti-inflammatory and autoimmune therapy) and spur the immune system to destroy endometrial lesions (immunomodulation). Early studies of certain immunotherapy drugs like anti-TNF agents that block inflammation show promise for reducing pain and shrinking lesions.

## Regenerative Medicine

Stem cell therapy and tissue engineering are exciting frontiers of regenerative medicine that could someday help restore normal pelvic anatomy and physiology for those with endometriosis. Scientists are working on using a woman's own stem cells to regrow healthy endometrial tissue, repair scar tissue damage from lesions, and restore fertility. While still largely experimental, regenerative techniques provide hope for more natural and permanent solutions.

Progress on these promising research fronts relies on continued funding, advocacy, and participation in clinical trials. By supporting organizations promoting endometriosis research and education, donating to researchers studying innovative treatments, and volunteering for ethically-conducted studies, you can play an active role in winning the battle against this disease. Together, we can build a future with better options for endometriosis management and, ultimately, a cure.[14]

---

[14] https://endometriosisassn.org/

https://www.endofound.org/

https://endometriosis.org/support/world-endometriosis-organisations-weo/

# 32

## CONCLUSION

Throughout the journey that is 'We Endo Warriors', we have traversed the landscape of endometriosis, a condition that affects millions of women worldwide. We've told the stories of the silent warriors, shedding light on the often-invisible battles they fight every day.

---

https://endomarch.org/about-endometriosis/who-we-are/

We've explored the science behind the condition, the current state of research, and the desperate need for more.

We wish to emphasize that while the journey with endometriosis is often marked by pain and challenges, it is also one of resilience and strength. The courage of Endo Warriors is unmatched, their spirit unbreakable.

The aim of this book was not only to educate but also to inspire action. We implore every reader to contribute what they can, be it spreading awareness, advocating for research funding, or lending a listening ear to those battling the condition.

The fight against endometriosis is a collective one. By standing together, supporting each other, we can transform the narrative around this condition from one of silent suffering to one of vocal victory.

Remember, every warrior's story is a beacon of hope, a testament to the human spirit's indomitable strength. As we conclude, let's carry these stories with us, let them inspire us to act, to fight, to conquer.

In the end, we're all in this together, walking side by side on the journey towards a world where endometriosis is no longer an invisible enemy, but a conquerable condition. Here's to every Endo Warrior - your courage lights the way."

# Summary of key points

Endometriosis is a disorder where tissue that usually lines the inside of the uterus grows outside it. This condition, while not externally visible, causes severe and debilitating pain, unusually heavy periods, and fertility challenges, often disrupting the daily lives of those affected.

Jetton goes on to highlight the unfortunate reality that many women suffer for years before receiving a proper diagnosis. The journey towards diagnosis is often marked by dismissals and misinterpretations, further compounding the frustration and despair faced by these individuals.

One of the key points Jetton emphasizes is the need for unity among endometriosis patients. She invites them to band together, labeling them as "warriors" in the battle against this disease. This sense of camaraderie and shared struggle is crucial in their journey.

In conclusion, Jetton underscores the crucial role of self-advocacy and education. Living with chronic pain necessitates a proactive approach in educating oneself and others about the realities of endometriosis. Addressing the lack of understanding and awareness about this condition is the first step towards combating it effectively.

We are calling on governments, health organizations, and private sectors to increase funding for research into endometriosis. By doing so, we can deepen our understanding of this complex condition, leading to more effective diagnostics and treatment options.

We also urge the development of new and improved medications that can truly alleviate the severe pain that endometriosis patients endure. This requires investment into pharmaceutical research dedicated to this cause.

Furthermore, we advocate for the prioritization of finding a cure for endometriosis. While managing symptoms is crucial, our aim should be to free women from this condition entirely.

Lastly, it's vital that we enhance the care provided to endometriosis patients. This includes better training for healthcare professionals to correctly diagnose and manage the condition, as well as providing comprehensive support services for those living with it.

Stand with us in our fight against endometriosis. Your support can make a significant difference in the lives of millions of women. Together, we can move from suffering in silence to finding solutions. Let's invest in a future where endometriosis is no longer an invisible illness, but a conquerable adversary.

# About the Author

Courtney Jetton, the author of "We Endo Warriors," is a passionate advocate for women's health, particularly in the area of endometriosis. She herself is a warrior in the battle against this debilitating condition, making her writing deeply personal and compelling.

Jetton's journey with endometriosis has been long and challenging, marked by misdiagnoses and dismissals. However, she has transformed her struggle into a source of strength, using it to educate others about this often-misunderstood illness.

Her book, "We Endo Warriors," is a testament to her resilience and commitment to raising awareness about endometriosis. She hopes to inspire other endometriosis patients to become advocates for their own health.

Jetton's writing is characterized by an intimate understanding of the physical and emotional toll of endometriosis, making her a powerful voice in the fight against this condition. With her honest and inspiring storytelling, she seeks to shed light on the invisible battle many women face, creating a sense of unity and empowerment among "Endo Warriors" worldwide.

www.weendowarriors.com

# Acknowledgments

I want to take a moment here and acknowledge all the beautiful souls who made this possible. Marissa Webb, my mom, who so graciously took time out of her busy day to give you her perspective of Endometriosis and what it does to loved ones. Alexander King, for being my rock over the years and forever pushing me to meet my goals. Both my mom and Alex have played vital roles in learning how to combat endometriosis in a more natural holistic manner. Ashlie Persilver, my dear friend who has been there since the beginning and encouraged me to write this book for all of you! I want to thank all the ladies who shared their stories and helped make this possible! It takes an incredible amount of strength and bravery to be willing to share your story with the world. Especially after being convinced that everything that is happening to you is all in your head by our ever so trusted medical professionals.

www.ingramcontent.com/pod-product-compliance
Lightning Source LLC
Chambersburg PA
CBHW051524020426
42333CB00016B/1774